SAMANTHA REDGRAVE

Flow

Self-care sessions for your menstrual, lunar,
life and seasonal cycles

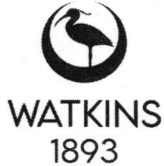

WATKINS
1893

Flow
Samantha Redgrave

First published in the UK and USA in 2025 by
Watkins, an imprint of Watkins Media Limited
Unit 11, Shepperton House, 83–89 Shepperton Road
London N1 3DF

enquiries@watkinspublishing.com

Commissioning Editor: Ella Chappell
Project Editor: Brittany Willis
Head of Design: Karen Smith
Design Concept: Sneha Alexander
Production: Uzma Taj

A CIP record for this book is available from the British Library

ISBN: 978-1-78678-883-2 (Paperback)
ISBN: 978-1-78678-884-9 (eBook)

10 9 8 7 6 5 4 3 2 1

MIX
Paper | Supporting
responsible forestry
FSC
www.fsc.org   FSC® C171272

Typeset by Lapiz
Printed and bound by CPI Group (UK) Ltd, Croydon, CR0 4YY

www.watkinspublishing.com

For Poppy-Jean and Elliot. You taught me the wisdom of divine timing, deep presence and unconditional love.

NOTE FROM THE AUTHOR

The mythical stories I share in this book are of European origins. As this is my heritage, I feel the only appropriate way to talk about cyclicality through the lens of folklore and ceremonies is to share those traditions I am familiar with and thus avoid potentially distorting or misrepresenting stories from non-European cultures. Please research folklore tales from your lineage as a way to ritualize your life. Understanding the flavourful history of your ancestors and the stories they would tell each other to develop meaningful and intimate connections is beautiful.

Please always use ethically sourced oils and check for any allergies and contraindications beforehand. Please research any contraindications in yoga and other exercises that may make certain movements inadvisable. And please always seek professional help when it comes to mental health support.

CONTENTS

BEGINNING

Modern life has become an endless conveyor belt of *doing*. We only need to speak to our friends to know how overworked, burnt-out, stressed and tired many of us feel. Women are drowning in over-productivity, often taking on too much. But why? To be better or more than? To be faster, to please others, to reach milestones? Or to avoid our thoughts and our truth, perhaps?

We can now live in a world where it's possible to do more than ever, but at what price? The message seems to be: if you want success and power, be consistent, productive and unchanging. Slow the ageing process, push through your body's insight, put aside your menstrual cycles and think little of the seasons and the moon. This is said only with love – I've done all of the above.

But this way was never "our" decision. Women are not meant to be perennial. We are dynamic, ever-changing beings that move with the cycles of time: life, seasonal, lunar and menstrual.

When we rewrite the script handed to us and return to a natural cyclicality we feel more in tune with our truth. Self-compassion, resilience, empowerment, joy and purpose effortlessly flow into our hearts and minds.

Flow invites you to come home. Together, here, we can carve out time to mindfully return to the natural rhythms of living.

I invite you to grow and rest with this cauldron of self-care practices, rituals, insights and tried-and-tested actionable tips.

I know that dipping out of life, with all its responsibilities, isn't an option for most of us. My intention here is to hold sacred the intricacies of the female experience, while understanding our collective overwhelm and the need for simplicity and manageability.

HOW TO USE THIS BOOK

Please navigate these pages according to your wisdom. If something doesn't click, doesn't feel right or goes against professional advice you have received, please side-step it. You are your greatest teacher, and you know your body best.

Even though I speak to women for the most part, using the she/her pronouns, I honour and welcome anyone with an interest in living in their flow, whatever that looks like for you. This book is for any woman, man or person who falls outside the gender binary standards, looking for self-care through cyclical living.

This book is split into four parts, each looking closely at the different cycles and how to invite them into our lives:

Part 1 looks at the **life cycle**, taking us through the four key archetypes of most women's lives, known as: Maiden, Mother, Wild Woman and Crone. We will explore ceremonies that celebrate your current archetype, with healing practices that allow you to become attuned to your inner self.

Part 2 focuses on the **seasonal cycle** – the flow of spring, summer, autumn and winter. I offer you rituals, practices and recipes that celebrate the season and the pagan festivals found within each.

Part 3 explores the **lunar cycle**, and how the four moon phases can influence our daily lives. You will discover spells and sigils to help you become more attuned to the moon.

Finally, in Part 4 we turn to the **menstrual cycle**, looking at physical, emotional and spiritual healing practices for every stage.

MY STORY

At the time of writing this book, I'm 43 and at the beginning of my Wild Woman or early autumn life cycle. I have two loving (and let's face it, sometimes exhausting) children aged 10 and 13. I've been in a relationship with their wonderful father for over 23 years. My family have taught me the importance of surrender, gifted me abundant love and laughter, brought old wounds to the surface and given me a heavy dose of resilience – all of which I am eternally grateful for.

Resilience served me well after a sarcoma cancer diagnosis in 2023 which, although deeply upsetting at the time, afforded me space to build a new way of living, one born from a more grounded form of self-growth and personal revelation. I now have the all-clear, and despite the life-changing diagnosis, I've kept my weird vibes.

This was not my first dip into the well of ill health. A two-year bout of chronic fatigue syndrome in my early 20s threw me off my graduate path and took me into the world of wellness and healing. It was here that I recovered – not only from CFS but from many "nice-girl" tendencies and perfectionist patterns (see more on this in Chapter 1).

As a result of this new fork in the road, I became a licensed hypnotherapist, using counselling, neuro-linguistic programming and hypno-analysis skills to help those struggling with emotionally related issues.

My career path expanded when another cyclical soul and I set up Aluna Moon. Together, we produced meditations and guided visualizations for platforms such as Insight Timer, YouTube and Audible. To the 100,000 lovelies in our Insight Timer community, I can't thank you enough for your continued support! I went on to produce wellbeing content for brands including *Happiful* Magazine, Counselling Directory, Twinkl and Moshi.

And this brings us to today. Through my life experiences, study and work, I discovered that cyclical living is part of who I am. Every day, I turn to my inner cycles to come closer to my truth. The lunar and yearly seasons remind me that I'm bound to a purpose and power far greater than myself, and remind me that I am worthy, whatever my output.

Your truth will be different to mine. *Flow* is an offering to walk alongside me each day, a little more sure-footed, with this guidance system of cyclical greatness.

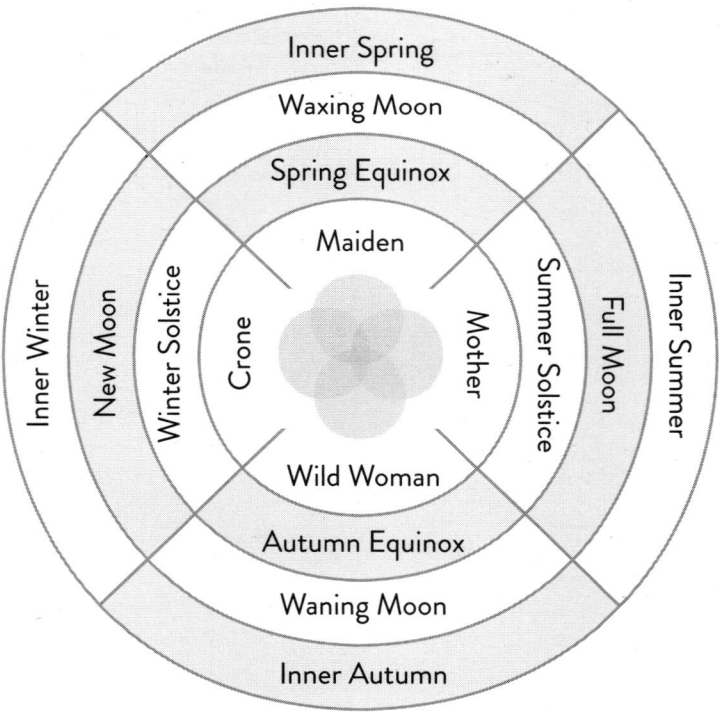

The four cycles: life, seasonal, lunar and menstrual

PART ONE

LIFE CYCLE

Our initiation into cyclical living begins with the seasons of life. Just as there are four phases of the year, four phases of the moon and four phases of the menstrual cycle, there are four phases, or seasons, of our life cycle.

Perhaps you're not yet sure of the lunar phases, or how to live in flow with your menstrual cycle, but one thing you will already know about is the natural ageing process. And it is natural, despite society telling us otherwise. As we flow from one life stage to another, we gain more beauty, insight and empowerment, transcending external and internal pressures to be anything other than ourselves.

Unfortunately, women have had hundreds of years of patriarchal conditioning telling us that the more women age, the less worthwhile we become. This is simply not true. As a collective, women have the strength to go against this.

If we're going to define these four stages of a woman's life cycle in archetypes (and please let's do as they're bloody amazing), we can term them as: Maiden, Mother, Wild Woman and Crone. These archetypes are often used in modern goddess spirituality, but please feel free to use any wording that fits for you.

ARCHETYPES AND PRONOUNS

Feminine pronouns are often used in connection to female archetypes and their representations. However, initiations of sacred strength, growth and empowerment are, of course, experienced by any gender. This is your journey, and your truth, so always use whatever language is good for you.

These archetypes are not as esoteric as they first seem. They help us make sense of the world and feel inspired in a way that doesn't get taken up with the usual limits of everyday being. We can work within the area of archetypes without getting mixed up in distorted or simplified versions of the female experience. These archetypes nest in the collective mind and our nervous systems, showing us the strengths and weaknesses of the female experience. We can see the archetypes as a doorway to deeper self-care and connection, and there are no limits when it comes to how to work with them.

These pages really are for everyone, no matter which life phase you're in. Let's begin with healing our younger years – our Maidens.

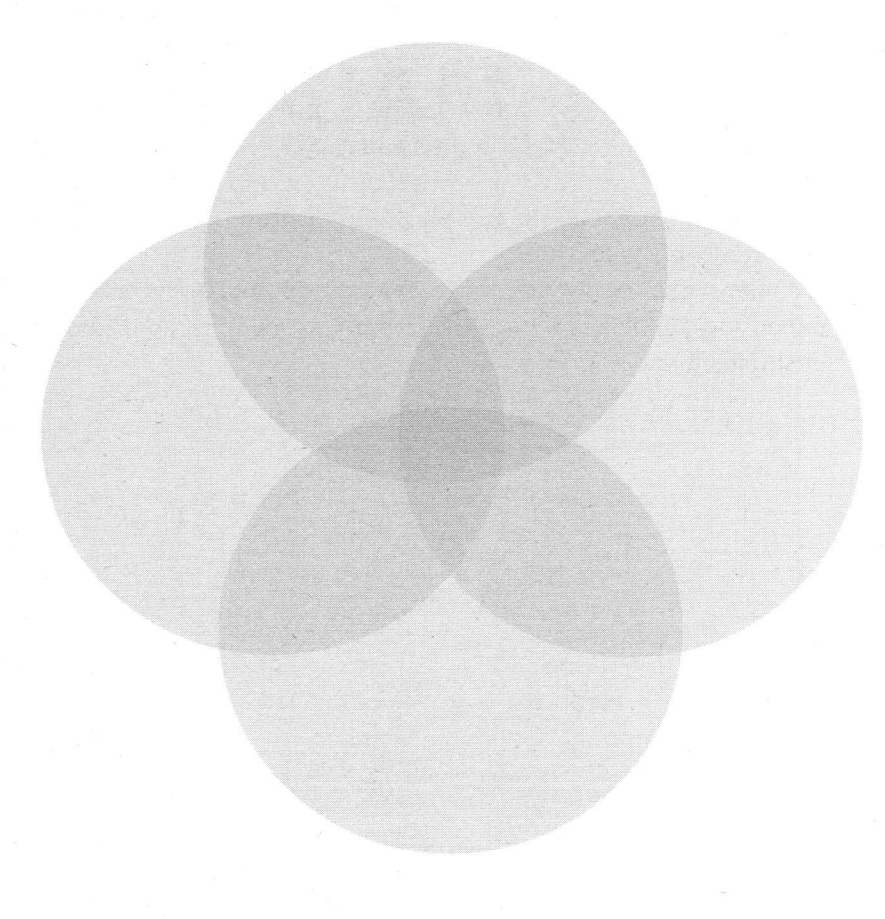

CHAPTER 1

THE MAIDEN

The Maiden stage usually begins during menarche (first period) and continues until the late 20s or so. I'm using the term "Maiden" as a nod to modern Wicca – don't worry, I'm not expecting you to throw your hair down a turret so your knight in shining armour can rescue you.

If you're in your Maiden cycle, you may feel like you have the world at your feet. Or you may feel the pressure of time to tick off a list of achievements and reach the many milestones society expects from you. The pressure to have it all (and be it all) feels, at times, palpable.

In the light, the Maiden archetype represents spring, new beginnings, hope, innocence, adventure, curiosity and limitless joy. She basks in the glimmers of life and feels a sense of wonder with each passing day.

The Maiden knows how to indulge her own fulfilment and rejects the need to be anything else. She is quite something! If this all sounds a bit romantic, in modern life these qualities look like optimism, potential, personal growth, courage and strength.

In literature and media, the Maiden has often been presented as a white, straight, able-bodied, cis-gender, repressed and submissive female. It's time we rewrite the narrative to portray the Maiden as something else. Maidens do not look a certain way, nor do they wait to be saved. Our Maiden is curious, potent, smart and stands strong.

There's always another side to the coin, and in the shadow, the Maiden can often be fearful, co-dependent and overly responsible. A Maiden might be defined as "too nice" or as trying "too hard". This is because she only feels good enough when others say so, causing her to "overcompensate". Perfectionism and people-pleasing become coping strategies for the Maiden. Is it any wonder that our Maidens become victims of "good girl" conditioning when we're taught to repress anger and put other people's feelings before our own? From the beginning, more is expected of us in terms of behaviour, hard work, responsibility and taking care of others. We, as women, are judged based on our output ... and on pretty much everything else, come to think of it.

The Maiden cycle is not about reinforcing the idea of a "damsel in distress", nor pigeonholing a woman's life experiences. We are simply exploring the symbolism behind what it's like to be a young female. And for some, it's hard-going.

Over-sexualization from others can also hold back the Maiden in many ways. Her natural, playful sensuality is sometimes hijacked by patriarchal objectification. This may cause the Maiden to separate from her body, living mostly in her mind. And it's this living in the mind that can bring about patterns of overthinking. As her body doesn't always feel safe, the Maiden tries to create spaces outside of herself to call home.

Modern-day Maidens are very likely to explore social media. It's normal to be curious about others, and how they live their lives, but this comparison culture, that's so embedded in our everyday (sometimes before we've even got out of bed!), is damaging to our care-free Maiden years. Emotional perfectionism, or needing life to be "better" or "happier", as well as jealousy, anxiety and low self-esteem that comes along too, seem to be some of the biggest fallouts from these online, synthetic images.

As I talk about the two sides of this life season archetype, where do you (or did you) sit, do you think? This book is never about blaming and shaming. I offer you a gentle curiosity as to how you experience your internal and external worlds, and how you might optimize your personal development journey to reach your fullest potential. Never give yourself a hard time! The prefrontal cortex, which is responsible for regulating our thoughts, actions and emotions, isn't even fully developed until the age of 25, so the Maiden cycle is all one big learning curve.

Feel free to use this chapter to re-evaluate this life season, embracing imperfection and growth, and letting go of the need to be "more". You can be your best self without layering on unrealistic or inflexible standards.

If you're in a later cycle of your life, you may wonder about your Maiden years and how you felt back then. Is there a Maiden wound? Did you hold back in some way? Are there any residual fears and shame associated with this time? If so, I suggest having a compassionate conversation with yourself to repair this hurt. This could be an internal chat, or you may want to journal your thoughts. You may ask yourself: what protective instincts were at play and what things did you learn? Validating your experience and reframing any negative inner dialogue can bring healing into any untrue beliefs you've been holding onto.

CHAKRA HEALING: STEP INTO YOUR POTENTIAL

This chakra-balancing exercise will help you move away from the shadow side of the Maiden, and into your true potential. If you're in another life phase and looking back at your Maiden era with some regrets or hurts, you can also try this exercise, perhaps imagining your younger self experiencing the benefits. We will focus on your sacral chakra or Svadhisthana, which is where your Maiden resides. It embodies self-worth, potential, sensuality and positive connections.

1. Find a safe space and make yourself comfortable. When you are ready, allow your eyes to close. Your sacral chakra is just below the navel, so bring your attention to this area.
2. Place your hand on your lower abdomen (your womb centre) and sit within this space for a while. This is a space of intimacy and creativity.
3. Take some deep abdominal breaths in through your nose, and into your sacral chakra. If you can, extend the inhale as long as feels comfortable, before releasing the breath fully on the exhale.
4. As you continue to breathe deeply, imagine a vibrant ball of orange light filling up this space. As you imagine this, feel your sacral chakra filling up with warmth and power. The light dissolves any limiting self-beliefs, flooding the space with creative potential.
5. Now, say to yourself some positive affirmations that feel good, such as:

> *I release the need to be perfect.*
> *I let go of unwanted fear.*
> *I embrace failure and growth.*
> *I create with courage.*
> *I express my needs.*
> *I deserve to thrive.*
> *I am pure potential.*

6. When you're ready, allow the image of the orange ball to fade away. Bring your breathing back to its normal pace, and allow your eyes to open.

THE MAIDEN AND MENARCHE

How we begin our Maidenhood odyssey can often be influenced by menarche. What was your experience of your first period like? How did you feel when you first saw your blood? I hope it was positive. Did your immediate circle react positively and warmly? Unfortunately, for many of my clients, this experience is imprinted with confusion, pain, dismissal or shame.

The collective narrative of menstruation is often one of "covering up" or discretion, at best. Advertising has gone to town on making sure we see periods as inconvenient or taboo. It's so odd to think that, not so long ago, a woman's period on TV was shown as blue liquid, not red, being poured into a sanitary towel.

Menarche is not something to be ashamed of, or an event to hide. Menarche is our initiation into something deeper. It's a rite of passage and a spiritual celebration of self-growth and empowerment. It forms how we take care of, and attend to, ourselves moving forward, partly outlining our identity as women.

Menstrual educator Lara Owen (see Further Reading) writes about the differences between how menarche is viewed in the Western world, compared with some indigenous cultures, in her pioneering book, *Her Blood Is Gold*. To sum up, she writes,

> "In the majority of cases, menarche remains an unritualized, uncelebrated, non-event, and as a society, we have a long way to go toward making the first period a time which supports a young girl and ushers her successfully into her adolescent years and indeed, her womanhood."

As you look back and wonder what your first period taught you, you may have wished it to be different somehow. One way to repair any lasting wounds from our first menstrual experience is to reclaim Maidenhood with a ritual. My years as a hypnotherapist have shown me the power of the mind to reframe an experience.

RECLAIM MENARCHE CEREMONY

If you're ready, and it feels right, let's begin this ceremony to heal and take back the power of menarche.

You will need:
- fire-proof bowl
- red candle
- lighter
- paper and a pen

1. Find a safe space and close your eyes. Revisit your first period in your mind's eye. Ask yourself, what does your first experience of bleeding feel like? Where are you when you first notice your period? Did you tell anyone that day, and if so, who?

2. Open your eyes and write down on your paper any messages your mind may have picked up about menstruation, positive and negative. Express anything you would like to let go of onto the paper, no matter how big or small. If you want to speak these feelings out loud as you write, feel free.

3. When you are finished, light the red candle, roll the paper up and set fire to it with the flame of the candle. Place it into the fire-proof bowl. As you witness the paper wither away, imagine that any negative feelings surrounding your first period are dissolving.

4. When the paper has burnt to dust, close your eyes. Imagine that your young self turns to look at you as your present self. Imagine that this younger you can now embrace this new body wisdom, as you say the following affirmation out loud:

"I release fear, I let go of shame, I honour my body."

5. Take a deep breath and allow these words to take root.

6. Open your eyes and return to your space with clarity, feeling renewed and refreshed.

Our first bleed focuses our awareness on the inner workings of the body, more specifically the womb. As we flow through our Maiden years, we build on this connection with ourselves. This self-relationship sets the pace for the way we treat and communicate with others. We learn much about the different parts of ourselves during this life stage, all without the weight of taking care of others. By the end of the Maiden apprenticeship, we now understand how we react, what goals we like to pursue and how we navigate challenges. These years prepare us for the responsibilities and gifts that await us in the Mother phase. Let's look at that next.

CHAPTER 2

THE MOTHER

The Mother archetype usually begins in your 30s, but, as always, there is no set model for our life seasons. You can access the Mother, or nurturer, archetype at any point in your life cycle, and there is no need to achieve certain life "milestones" to create space for this kind of self-development.

To make it super-clear: you don't need to be a Mother or want to have children to work with this archetype. This archetype is all about feeling the love for others and for the world around you. It's not so much about self, which is felt more deeply in the Maiden years. And it's definitely not about the oh-so-capitalist idea of being a "good" person by doing way too much for other people. Don't worry, I'm not suggesting here that you dash around looking after everyone else, giving up your own desires and dreams.

The Mother phase of your life cycle is about community connection and healing. This involves nurturing yourself as much as nurturing others. This is a stage of life when things come to full bloom – whether that's relationships, work or family life. It's an unconditional kind of love that isn't reliant on, or regulated by, circumstances and achievements.

Don't be fooled by any stereotypical matriarch figures seen in films; this archetype can be as fierce as she can be soft. The Mother energy is about becoming resilient in life and tending to a greater strength within. Big growth happens in this cycle, and we can't help bringing everyone else along for the ride (in the most well-intentioned way, of course!). And it's this self-development, spurred on by the Mother's ability to reframe setbacks, that gives way to success and flourishing creativity, for yourself and those around you.

I love the way Clarissa Pinkola Estés talks about the transformation from Maiden to Mother (see Further Reading), through the lens of her modern-ancient endurance tale, *The Handless Maiden*, in *Women Who Run With The Wolves:*

> "The teaching of endurance occurs all through nature. The pads of wolf's pups' paws are soft as clay when the pups are born. It is only the ranging, the roaming, the treks on which their parents take them that toughen them up ... They are toughening up the sweet little spirit, investing with strength and resilience."

In this, we see the arc of the female journey and the spiritual strength needed as we grow in years. The Maiden has been building toward something through the adventures (and misadventures) of everyday life. Along the way, many lessons were learnt and many dreams were conceived. This well-earned resilience fosters an initiation into the Mother. Now, it is not just about "self-development" but about sharing our stories with those who need it. We're supposed to transform with every life phase, embodying the sacred gifts and challenges of each.

How does the Mother archetype manifest? On good days, the Mother archetype represents summer, coming into bloom, abundance, fertility or potency, an initiator of change and a trustee of gorgeous generosity. In modern-day life, this looks like compassion, protection, tenderness, resilience, creativity and empathy. This joyful side of the Mother can be energizing to be around.

In the shadow, the Mother archetype can forget her way if she doesn't have a creative outlet, losing a sense of identity in the quest to be only of service to others. In everyday life, this can take the form of being taken advantage of, feeling uninspired, finding it difficult to say no, or feeling overly responsible for others. This may mean you feel guilty for not doing enough for those around you, or lack the boundaries needed to keep your relationships healthy. Taking on board other people's worries can make you feel exhausted and overwhelmed.

CHAKRA HEALING: MEET YOUR WELL-RESTED WOMAN

The exercise will help you move away from the shadow side of the Mother, who is overwhelmed by the needs of others. Instead, you can experience a lovely moment of self-compassion. If you're in another life phase, you can still experience the restful benefits of this chakra-balancing exercise. Your heart chakra or Anahata is the star here and it's all about connection, love and feeling at peace with your true self.

1. Find a safe space and make yourself comfortable. When you are ready, allow your eyes to close. Bring your attention to your heart chakra (the centre of your chest) for a few moments.

2. Place your hand on your heart chakra and sit within a space of self-love for a while.
3. Take some deep breaths in and out through your nose. Imagine your inhale expands from the centre of your heart, through to your fingers. As you exhale, relax back toward the centre of your chest. Continue this heart-to-hand breathing for a few moments.
4. As you continue to breathe in this way, imagine an orb of green light filling up your heart space with love, dissolving any resentment and guilt.
5. Now, say to yourself some affirmations that feel good, such as:

I am deserving of rest.
It's OK to say no and have good boundaries with others.
I choose to be kind to myself.
I allow myself to accept compliments.
I have the courage to overcome setbacks.
I am a source of loving creativity.
I am pure, lasting love.

6. When you are ready, bring your breathing back to its normal pace, and allow your eyes to flutter open. Great work!

MOTHERHOOD

Creation comes in many forms. Showing the world what we've got to offer may come from our life experiences and lessons, and it may also come about through the journey of Motherhood. There will be some of you reading this page who are parents, so this is a good time to reflect on your Motherhood experiences while we delve into all the corners of this archetype. If you're not a parent, you can still experience the benefits of the ceremony later in this chapter. It's an opportunity to reflect on how you were raised and the type of relationship you have, or had, with your Mother.

How do you experience Motherhood? That's a big question to ask, I know. What parts bring you the most happiness? What do you find most difficult? What do you feel good about in terms of the way you parent? What might you like to learn to do differently? Perhaps you've found Motherhood to be an easy ride, or perhaps it's felt really hard-going at times. It's certainly a life initiation, one full of gains and losses.

It also may be worth reflecting on the birth(s) of your child(ren). What was it like for you? What was your postpartum period like? Were you supported? Take some time thinking, or journaling, about your entry into Motherhood and give yourself much love and praise for the way you handled this experience.

My first birth was long, slow and arduous; a complete shock that took me much time to process, both physically and emotionally. The second was fierce and beautiful, and I can only describe it as a complete "handing over" of myself. For me, those early years of Motherhood were a blur of joy, pain and everything in between.

Despite birth feeling bloody awful for some of us, it's these tests of endurance, I think, that can engrave our surrender to something greater than ourselves. Lisa Marchiano (see Further Reading) talks about the opportunity that Motherhood brings to psychological growth in her book, *Motherhood:*

"Motherhood, with its intense physical and emotional extremes, is a crucible in which we are tested and altered. Outdated parts of personality are melted away, and new structures are forged ... Motherhood is the ultimate confrontation with yourself. Whatever is there to discover at the bottom of your soul, whether dross or treasure, Motherhood will help you find it."

I've certainly found Motherhood to be a rollercoaster. How we parent can, of course, be influenced by how our caregivers raised us. And how our Mothers tended to us is, in turn, dictated by their own upbringing and childhood experiences. When we have unhelpful or painful experiences growing up, it can impact the way we speak to ourselves, how we develop relationships and how we deal with life's struggles in adulthood. Often patterns are repeated through generations and this can be known as a "Mother wound".

Mother wounds

A Mother wound doesn't have to be anything sinister, although sometimes this is the case. It can simply be not having your needs met, and this can make you feel dismissed or inadequate in some way. These feelings can come to a head when we're "confronted" with ourselves, when having our own children. Mother wounds can then play out in our everyday lives and often show up in feelings of "not-enough", affecting the way we parent our children.

When we're brought up by Mothers or caregivers who are "unconscious" of their behaviour, they can prevent us from connecting to our hearts and deepest selves. The inability to connect with our Mother in ways that we perhaps needed can mean we suffer emotionally.

This Mother wound can look like many things, such as criticism, narcissism, perfectionism, abuse, detachment, resentment, anger, body issues, addiction, low self-esteem, mental health conditions, or something else that I haven't covered here that feels relevant for you and your circumstances.

Working with a Mother wound symbolically can be a gentle way to work through any hurt you have experienced. Please do seek out help from a professional if you're struggling with any of the issues talked about in this chapter.

MOTHER WOUND CEREMONY

Here, we shine a gentle light on any generational patterns you have experienced, and allow a space of healing and self-soothing to take root.

Only take part in this ceremony when you have the right kind of space; by this I mean when you feel emotionally ready and have a place where you won't be disturbed. As always, please listen to your intuition.

You will need:
- pen
- paper
- candle, of your choosing

1. Write down some of the "not-enough" feelings you experience. This might include the harsh ways you speak

to yourself. You could also note how this manifests in your relationship with others, including your children.

2. Now, write down the things you want to feel next to it. For example, if you wrote, "I belittle my achievements and think other people are better than me", you may want to hear something like, "My self-worth is not dependent on how I perform. I am lovable just as I am".

3. Now, close your eyes and imagine a miniature version of your childhood self. You may like to imagine that little figure in front of you. If this is difficult, imagine a favourite colour or shape instead.

4. Tell younger you all the things you wrote down that they may like to hear. Tell them, in your own words, that you/ they are enough. You may like to hug them.

5. Allow your younger self to feel loved unconditionally.

6. When you have spent as long as you feel is right here, come away from this image with love in your heart.

7. With your eyes open, light the candle. As you watch it burn, imagine the Mother wound melting.

8. When you're ready, say out loud,

> *"I create a safe relationship with myself. I choose a different path for the generations to come. I am enough."*

These words will help you claim your generational gifts and let go of ancestral trauma.

9. Before you leave, take a deep breath. Know that you are more than your wounds; you are powerful!
10. Come back to the space when you're ready, with a renewed feeling of strength.

The Mother energy brings a sense of responsibility. Whether you are working through maternal wounds, looking after a child or sharing your creativity and knowledge with the world, there is a level of commitment needed to "carry off" this phase. Walking the tightrope of self-care and compassion for others isn't easy. We need to give, but not too much. It's a challenge that will linger as we cross over into the Wild Woman years, where the focus returns to personal needs and desires. Different to before, we learn to speak our truth and evolve our power in a way that's only possible with the teachings of the Maiden and Mother.

CHAPTER 3

THE WILD WOMAN

This is when life starts to get juicy. The Wild Woman archetype usually takes to the stage in a woman's 40s, but the timings, as always, aren't fixed. In goddess spirituality, there is very little mention of the Wild Woman archetype, centring on the Maiden, Mother and Crone chapters of a woman's life cycle. She was hidden, and still is today, to some extent. In today's society, the Wild Woman is often feared or even rejected. In more recent years, this archetype has been resurrected, and she is an absolute powerhouse!

How does the Wild Woman archetype manifest? In alignment, she represents spontaneity and untamed sexual expression. This doesn't look chaotic; instead, she has good boundaries and understands her true value. The Wild Woman archetype speaks her truth and can defend both herself and others, sharing much-needed honesty. She's learnt the power of discipline, understanding the importance of being active to get things done and to do them well.

At the same time, there is something very witchy about this medicine woman, who feels the rhythms of life in a way that the other archetypes, perhaps, do not. In everyday life, empowered midlife can show up as authenticity, sexual freedom, self-reliance, revolution, persistence and courage. Can you tell this is my favourite? Hello, me at 43!

As with every life archetype, there is a shadow side. When it's overcast, the Wild Woman can slip into toxic independence. There are many variations of this: for example, the Wild Woman can become so consumed with her desires and goals that she ends up forgetting her vulnerability, becoming annoyed when anyone gets too attached or reminds her of her emotional wounds. In modern life, this can materialize as avoidant attachment, irritability and resistance to embracing any difficulties she's faced in life.

As with nature, wildness can descend into destruction, so the autumn years can feel like a bit of a wrecking ball for some, especially if that wildness doesn't have a healthy, creative outlet (see page 15). Anger at the world and its expectations, coupled with fluctuating hormones, may leave some of you feeling resentful or anxious. Some women reject their wilder woman altogether, burying any underlying feelings of wanting things to be different or freer. This can trickle down into feelings of disappointment and regret.

When we keep ourselves back, we unfortunately deny ourselves the resources we need to unshackle from long-standing demands and responsibilities. It's restricting, paralyzing and like holding back a raging river within.

And so, a woman's 40s can feel a bit like a crossroads. It *can* be a potent time of self-discovery, but inhibitions and expectations can pull a woman back from "undimming" her true authority. The well-trodden path of going about things in the way we're used to, or required to, can feel like the easier, and perhaps the only, route to take during midlife.

Clarissa Pinkola Estés talks about the Wild Woman (see Further Reading) within us all, and how for some of us our true feminine power remains imprisoned:

> "Somehow many women are able to maintain themselves in a captured state, but they live a half-life or a quarter-life or even an nth-life. They manage, but may become bitter to the end of their days. They may feel hopeless, and often, like a babe who has cried and cried with no human aid forthcoming, they may become deathly silent and despairing. Fatigue and resignation follow. The cage is locked."

Taking the other fork in the road, the path of the wilder woman, can erupt in a yearning for something deeper. Being able to express your needs, perhaps in a way that you haven't been able to access before, is the crowning glory of the unrestricted woman in pursuit of her truth.

Let's now take some time together, to surrender to this free spirit and attend to the Wild Woman within, with this chakra healing practice:

CHAKRA HEALING: UNLEASH YOUR INNER VOICE

If you're in your Wild Woman era, you can use this practice to encourage a more uninhibited version of yourself. Your throat chakra, or Vishuddha, is the headliner for this healing session, and it's all about purpose, expression, authenticity and integrity. Opening your throat chakra encourages these qualities. Even though this practice is about potency, it's a grounded version, encouraging you to speak your truth in a way that considers others.

1. Find a safe space and make yourself comfortable. When you are ready, gently allow your eyes to close. As your Wild Woman resides in your throat chakra, bring your awareness to your neck for a few moments.
2. Give yourself permission to let go of any tightness in your body, especially your throat and neck area.
3. Take some long breaths in and out through your nose. Feel yourself slow down. Notice the cool breath moving down your throat and release the warmer breath fully on the exhale.
4. As you breathe in this way, imagine a sphere of blue light taking up space in the centre of your throat. Imagine the blue light expanding and rising to your mouth, ears and the back of your neck. As you imagine this, feel your chakra coming alive with purpose and into a place of surrender and knowing. The light dissolves any limits.
5. Say to yourself some affirmations that feel powerful, such as:

> *My voice is important and heard by others.*
> *I shine brightly and ask for what I need.*
> *I speak with honesty and kindness.*
> *I hold space for strength and vulnerability.*
> *I listen to my potent intuition.*
> *I am my true self.*

6. Bring your breathing back to its normal pace, and allow your eyes to flutter open when you're ready.

THE WILD WOMAN AND PERIMENOPAUSE

We need to talk about hormones here. During your 40s, there's a fluctuation in your hormone levels, which brings with it all sorts of emotional and physical changes. "Menopause" itself is a one-day event, which usually occurs in a woman's early 50s, 12 months after their last period. The years (ranging from two to ten) leading up to this are known as perimenopause. Did you know that over 90 per cent of women have perimenopausal symptoms during this time? Symptoms can include palpitations, anxiety, muscle and joint aches, hot flushes, fatigue, brain fog, and changes to skin, hair and periods.

NOURISH YOURSELF

If you're looking to alleviate any symptoms associated with perimenopause, or to simply to look after yourself during this time, you may like to read *The Happy Menopause* (see Further Reading) by Jackie Lynch. She talks about the value of nutrition in supporting the years leading up to menopause such as eating fewer refined carbohydrates and sugary foods, and eating foods rich in vitamins B, and C, phytoestrogens and magnesium.

There are emotional repercussions to perimenopause. Many women feel written off, especially during their late autumn years, feeling relegated by society and dismissed by negative stereotypes about ageing. This super-unfriendly dialogue surrounding midlife can happen in the workplace as well as within relationships, making it difficult for women to own their full power. This can make women experiencing perimenopause feel angry, and rightly so. The problem is that society doesn't like "angry" women, but it's this rage, or sacred rage as many spiritual folks call it, that propels change and births us into a place of transformation.

Midlife is feeling the fire within. It's getting to know ourselves outside of the "good girl" conditioning (see page 6), and it's obeying the urge to embody our full selves without shame. But we live in a world that doesn't support this Wild Woman transition, or worse, ruptures it. In this world, how can we be truly faithful to our truth, and get fired up by personal growth and revolution?

This prejudice started long ago. In Ancient Greece, the hormonal changes during perimenopause and menstruation were known as "hysteria". This hysteria came out of the idea of the "wandering womb", which according to male physicians, would cause tremors and anxiety in women. When I say wandering, the uterus was literally believed to climb up the body like some sort of devouring animal, causing chest pain and even suffocation. And yet, this word persists.

Women, throughout time, and still in many places around the word today, are expected to conform. Historically, many wild women who asserted themselves to the patriarchal forces were locked up or condemned for witchcraft. Given the patriarchal past and the domination and exploitation of women, is it any wonder how daunting it is for us to say "no" to others? And why do so many women find it agonizing to say "yes" to themselves?

During perimenopause, we have the chance to get to know and express our anger and our hurtful conditioning, but we get fobbed off as "going through the change" or being "hormonal".

It's time we come together to unleash the Wild Woman within and put our needs at the top of the pile. Being aware is the first step, so we're doing great! The second step is dedicating well-deserved time to actively heal. So, let's do that now.

REWILDING CEREMONY

This exercise is about serving our deepest desires by shedding outdated, divisive messages of fear and disconnection. A bold ceremony for a big archetype.

You will need:
- paper
- pen
- candle, of your choosing
- fire-proof bowl

1. Write down on your paper some of the things you're angry about or some of the things that have held you back. Allow those feelings to move through your body, down through your arm, and into your hand as you write.
2. When you've finished, roll up the paper. Light the candle, and burn the paper, over the fire-proof bowl. Watch the flames devour the ways you have been made to feel less than, or fearful.
3. Drop the paper into the bowl. As you watch the smoke rise, say out loud:

"I am wild like the moon, the earth, the sun and my dreams. I honour my Wild Woman within, with tenderness and love."

4. Take a moment to embrace your feet, with both hands, and say, "I will stay grounded in my truth and walk the right path for me".
5. Now bring your hands to your stomach and say, "I obey my intuition and gently hold space for my sacred feelings of rage".
6. Touch your ears and say, "I listen to, and respect, my innermost desires for the greater good".
7. Gently place your hands over your eyes and say, "I see the world clearly and seek the truth".
8. Bring your hands to the top of your head and say, "I am connected to my most authentic self and the world around me".
9. Come back to the space when you're ready with a feeling of grounded wildness, ready to take on the world!

The Wild Woman looks for new ways of speaking. She realizes that her words are valuable and that she now needs them to be heard. The Maiden's potential has evolved into potency and the Mother's compassion converts into creative fire. Guided by the need for change, this priestess lives in alignment with a new belief system, one that is less bound by the expectations of others. This wildness within is needed as we journey into the trials and blessings of the Crone years.

CHAPTER 4

THE CRONE

The Crone archetype usually begins in a woman's 50s, during the postmenopausal years. This life season is often our longest life phase, and a time when a woman can live to the full, according to her terms. With the fall of oestrogen and the end of a woman's menstrual journey, we can call this our life season of winter. But we can also see it as a second spring, representing a renewal of self and a moving away from nurturing others, to nurturing the self.

Our Westernized culture has diminished the authority of the experienced woman, revering instead the charm of Maidenhood and the promised land of timeless youth. Ageism has become so embedded in our bones that we barely even notice it on a daily basis. Instead of putting this wise matriarch at the centre of the community, we discriminate against older women, believing that the Crone has somehow passed her sell-by date in terms of purpose and usefulness. It's no surprise that we become seduced by the prospect of looking younger. But "keeping up" with youthfulness goes against the inherent virtue of the Crone, who has the opportunity to free herself from the heavy demands of others. Instead, this is a time to focus on the badass wisdom she's been cultivating through many years of impressive life experience.

What do you think of when you hear the word "Crone"? The word Crone derives from "crown", symbolizing the halo of light circling a woman of maturity and wisdom. Yet we tend to think of "old hags" or other negative words or imagery. Writer Mona Chollet (see Further Reading) talks about how we need to shatter the image of the old hag in her book, *In Defence of Witches*:

> "The disqualification of women's experience represents an immense loss to and mutilation of our collective knowledge. Urging women to change as little as possible and censoring the signs of their maturing means locking them into a debilitating schema. A moment's thought reveals the insane idealization entailed by our cult of youthfulness."

The witch hunts throughout history propelled this dislike or discrimination of the older woman. The hag, who didn't partake in the usual customs of society, was no longer of childbearing age and was most definitely more wilful than younger, more obedient women. She was seen as a bit of an anarchist, and back then, anything feared was to be destroyed.

But as a collective, we can revitalize the potency of Cronehood, remembering the incredible gifts and insights of the Crone, once more. Who is this cosmic medicine woman and what are her strengths, exactly?

The Crone is an advice-giver with a deep presence and wisdom that can only come from really tasting life. She is the darkness of the new moon, the sharp and unrestrained breath of winter and the wondrous and complete cycle of life. The Crone energy makes me feel very poetic! In everyday living,

Crone energy can take the shape of mentoring, integrity, intuition, discernment and sagacity.

Sharon Blackie (see Further Reading) writes about the ways women can bloom, during what is often seen as a time of decline, in her book, *Hagitude*. Blackie explores the unhealthy stereotypes we hold of ageing women in today's society:

> "Truth is, there is no clear image of enviable female elderhood in the contemporary cultural mythology of the West; it's not an archetype we recognise anymore. In our culture, old women are mostly ignored, encouraged to be inconspicuous or held up as objects of derision and satire ... In our more distant past, as of course in many indigenous cultures today, female elders were respected, and had important and meaningful roles to play."

With each archetype, there is an unhealed side. In the shadow, the Crone may feel emotionally cut off or "bitter", especially if she feels unseen or "put out to pasture". Sometimes, the Crone may overcompensate for this social disregard by taking on a "know-it-all" attitude as a way to "manually" elevate the self.

How you cross this rite of passage may at least partly depend on how you experienced your maternal line stepping into their Cronehood. It may be worth reflecting on this as you wonder about the shadow aspects of becoming a Crone, and how your views on getting older may prevent full-bodied wisdom from coming to fruition. Let's explore this now.

CHAKRA HEALING: INVITING INNER WISDOM

Use this exercise to call on your inner wisdom whenever you need a good dose of self-trust. If you're postmenopausal and feel restricted in your journey of being authentically you, use this chakra healing session to bring about a feeling of perception and harmony. The Ajna chakra, associated with the Crone archetype, nests in the middle of the eyebrows, parallel to the pineal gland, which is a pea-sized gland located in the centre of the head. It is known as the seat of the soul or the third eye.

1. When you have the right space and it's safe to relax, close your eyes and bring your awareness to the spot in the middle of your eyebrows.
2. As you breathe, notice how this area feels for you. Is there any tension? Do you feel relaxed here?
3. Now, imagine a purple light entering this space, opening up your third eye chakra. The orb of purple continues to grow as you breathe deeply and slowly.
4. Say to yourself some affirmations that feel powerful, such as:

   I have a clear mind and can see the truth easily.
   I am flexible to the natural changes that life brings.
   I am connected to a higher spiritual insight.
   I make decisions that support me.
   I give helpful guidance to others when it's needed.
   I am a source of intuitive wisdom.

5. Bring your breathing back to its usual rhythm, and allow your eyes to open gently when you're ready.

THE CRONE AND POSTMENOPAUSE

Menopause occurs due to a decline in oestrogen, usually between the ages of 45–55. Symptoms of postmenopause may include a loss of libido, vaginal dryness, difficulty concentrating, changes in body shape, headaches and difficulty sleeping. The average age for a black woman to experience the end of their periods is two years younger than the average age for a white woman, and black women may endure symptoms for longer. According to a 2022 study by Study of Women's Health Across the Nation (SWAN), structural racism may be at the root of these differences due to the care and treatment offered.

EARLY MENOPAUSE

Early menopause is when a woman's periods stop permanently before the age of 45. This could be due to a hysterectomy or premature ovarian failure perhaps related to an autoimmune disease, infection, cancer treatments or family history.

Postmenopause can be a vulnerable time for some women, especially when it comes to assessing our lives to this point. Often, we're presented with a catalogue of milestones (education, partner, children, travel, career …) to reach in perfect chronological order during our Maidenhood. When we haven't managed to collect all those badges of achievement by the time we reach our Crone years, we may look back with a sense of regret or failure.

The truth is that the present moment is all we have. When we live our lives surrendered to the here and now, we reduce the stress of menopause but also tap into a deeper meaning of life. We might have more time to enjoy and romanticize the little things that life brings. We can invite new practices into our everyday lives, such as mindfulness, walking in nature, cooking healthy foods, exercise, trying new things and, most importantly, having fun. A quick note on weight-bearing exercise: it is great for strength, bone density and posture. Do try it!

When we turn "inner winter" on its head, the Crone stage is actually a time of renewal and growth. There is nothing to prove to the world and no f**ks given! What a relief this is, after decades of being locked up in a capitalist pressure-cooker of doing and achieving. Instead, you can focus on your internal satisfaction and healing, naturally mentoring others to feel and be the same.

As author and artist Miranda Gray (see Further Reading) says of the Crone archetype in her book *Red Moon*:

"She has continuous access to the inner world dimension of life which is only accessible to the menstrual woman once a month."

CRONING CEREMONY

Claiming the ancient wisdom of the Crone with excitement and joy can be carried out alone or with a group of like-minded women who can witness this beautiful rite of passage. And as with any hero's journey, there are three stages to this journey of self-exploration: leaving behind, change and embodiment. Our croning ritual will centre on this same passage of initiation.

You will need:
- walking boots
- bag for gathering
- paper
- pen
- empty jar
- small mirror

LEAVING BEHIND

1. When it's time to Crone up, put on your walking boots and go for a long walk in nature, perhaps somewhere you haven't been before.
2. As you are walking, take some time to reflect on the past years as a Maiden, Mother and Wild Woman. Think about the changes you have made and the many lessons learnt; the times you have loved and lost, the moments you took a risk, the challenges you have overcome, the joyous days and the painful times. This is a mindful walk of deep self-discovery, so allow yourself to feel all the feels, rooting down into the earth beneath you.
3. While walking, collect some leaves, petals and twigs. Willow branches are great! You will need enough to make a Crone crown.
4. As you return home, reflect on how you feel ready to leave your former identity behind and excited about claiming this new chapter of your life.

CHANGE

1. When home, make a nature crown. You can use elastic, floristry wire or a headband as your base, wrapping, weaving or gluing (a hot glue gun works well) the stems and other natural items.
2. Next, take your paper and pen, and write down the amazing virtues and qualities you are ready to claim. It's great to make these as specific and heartfelt as possible, such as intuition, knowledge and confidence.
3. When you have written down everything you need, put the paper in the empty jar.
4. If you are performing this ceremony with others, ask your fellow goddesses to write down the strengths they witness in you. Place the slips of paper into your jar/s when finished.

EMBODIMENT

1. If you have made one, this is a lovely time to wear your nature crown.
2. Look at yourself in the mirror as you read each note out loud. If you are with others, the same process occurs without the mirror; others will witness beautifully the transformation and embodiment of your Cronehood.
3. As you read each note, feel your words flowing through your body, really absorbing the messages of renewal and awakening.
4. If you would like, read out the poem below, either in front of the mirror or to your fellow women. This completes the ceremony and activates the final stage of crowning your

Cronehood. You may prefer to pen your own words of initiation, and please do!

Here, I surrender many things,
The push to please.
The urgency to be right.
The need to be one thing or another.

Instead, I tend to my truth,
An everyday spaciousness.
A life fused with endless possibilities.
A perception that transcends worn-out limits.

Leaving, I return with a crown,
A crest of undying wisdom.
A queenship of unconditional love.
A prize of many losses and more gains.
I am the Crone.

The soul's soil is enriched with the stories from our Maiden, Mother and Wild Woman years. Before walking the terrain of the Crone, we had to wait for all the felt and forgotten parts of ourselves to "arrive". Now, your experiences and lessons fuse with your everyday, living moment to moment. This allows you to connect the dots in the chaos and hand down this wisdom to those who need it. Cronehood supports you to live as you wish. So, what do you want?

PART TWO

SEASONAL CYCLE

Take a moment, loves.

We are about to widen our cyclical journey by talking about the seasons. Before we do, I would love to know how you feel about the different seasons of the year. Which one/s do you feel the most alignment with? Winter, spring, summer or autumn? Perhaps you feel most at home with the warmth of the sun on your skin, or maybe you prefer the cozy, quieter months?

Each season brings a set of unique strengths and opportunities. When we come closer to understanding the gentle shifts of the year, we can flow easily with each season's changeful energies. Change is good, but sometimes in this 24/7, unforgiving and fast-moving world, it can look more like a never-ending "chase". We can yearn for the kind of productiveness that's reserved only for the lighter months.

If, like me, you fall into the trap of hunting down the "before and after" – whether that's in relation to what we've achieved, the things we do, the relationships we have or how we look – we can forget to lean into nature and the changing seasons. Associating with the earth, especially when it comes to the peaceful letting-go processes of the colder months, gives us a full, expanded human experience.

The seasons are our biggest teacher: patience, resilience, surrender, abundance and rebirth can all be learnt through the relationship we have with our natural surroundings. We can never fully return to the way our ancient communities would have embodied the natural rhythms of the earth, but we can live intentionally and more in time with the seasons.

SEASONAL LIVING AND CLIMATE CHANGE

Just as the seasons can support us, we can support our seasons. Milder winters, weather extremes, ecological disasters and climate change are very real. This means many of us can experience eco-anxiety and a sense of hopelessness about the future of the planet.

More than ever, we need to stay connected to the natural world, and be actionable when it comes to treading the earth a little more lightly. Seek out others who also want a better world, and take steps to help. For example, you might want to avoid fast fashion, ditch the car when possible or make some changes to how you eat, such as growing your own food, shopping seasonally or eating less meat. These will help to take control of your own carbon footprint.

Next, let's seek to honour the seasonal cycle with a witchy-esque tour of the year. The Wheel of the Year gives us the perfect terrain to ritualize our connection with the earth.

Together, we will travel through those first, sweet promises of spring, into the have-it-all energies of summer, then call back home our outer selves in autumn, in preparation for the quieter energies of the winter months. In these self-care sessions, we will look at how to optimize each season of the year, including how to ritualize the season's strengths, and let go of any self-limiting beliefs that crop up with each nudge of the wheel.

You can begin this section in whatever season you may find yourself in today. Each sacred season gives us an opportunity to move into a place of healing and belonging. And in this modern-day world, we could all do with a heavy-duty dose of feeling supported by something bigger than ourselves.

WHEEL OF THE YEAR

The Wheel of the Year consists of eight celebrations or sabbats, each of which connects us to the cycles of nature and Mother Earth. The continuous passage of time is symbolized through the image of a wheel to mark the changing seasons. The date of when each season starts, depends on whether you live in the northern or southern hemisphere.

Event	Northern hemisphere	Southern hemisphere
Imbolc	1 February	1 August
Ostara (Spring Equinox)	21 March	21 September
Beltane	1 May	31 October
Litha (Summer Solstice)	21 June	21 December
Lammas	1 August	1 February
Mabon (Autumn Equinox)	21 September	21 March
Samhain	31 October	1 May
Yule (Winter Solstice)	21 December	21 June

Note: The exact dates of the Wheel of the Year may differ according to the year.

The Wheel of the Year, often celebrated by modern-day pagans, is a relatively new system designed by the pioneers of Wicca. Our ancestors relied on their connection to the natural world to understand when to plant and harvest. Ancient communities understood the inherent link between divinity and nature and revered the sacred significance of the earth, and the Wheel of the Year honours this.

The shift from earth-based worship to organized religion has seen a spiritual disruption from nature for many. It seems that seasonal living is relegated in favour of productivity and consistency (another product of capitalism). It's now expected that our output should be the same all year round, with seasons seemingly fusing into one. I believe this adds to our collective stress and tells us that rest is something to feel remorseful about. Getting to know the different seasons and points of the year through practices and rituals is a truly special way to understand ourselves better. Simply put: our inner seasons mirror the outer seasons.

No matter how hard society tries to talk us into a linear "rational" way of living, we have an instinctual knowledge about the cycles of life and how to live in tune with nature. The Wheel of the Year is one lens to honour the external seasons, helping us to see ourselves in nature, more fully. Note that the dates in the wheel below are the Northern hemisphere ones.

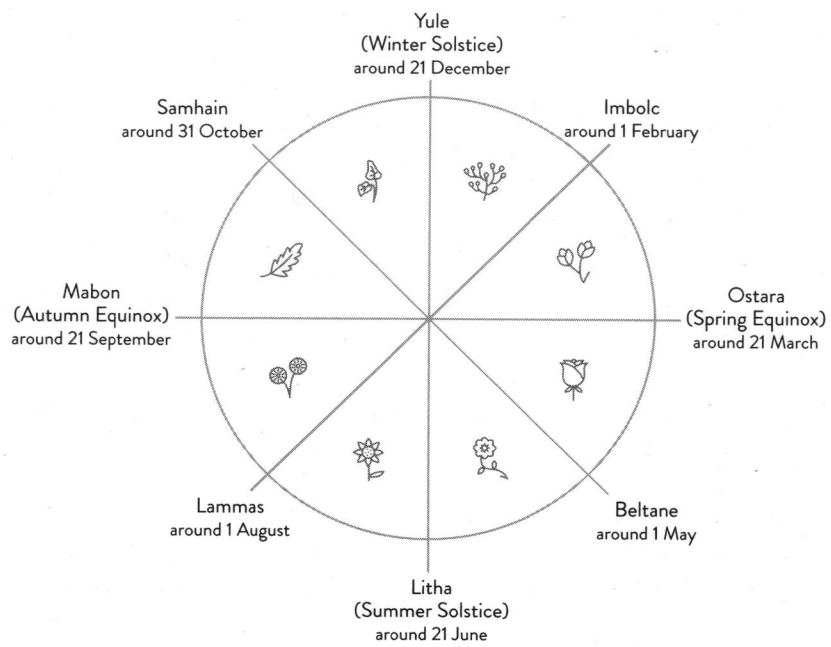

Yule
(Winter Solstice)
around 21 December

Samhain
around 31 October

Imbolc
around 1 February

Mabon
(Autumn Equinox)
around 21 September

Ostara
(Spring Equinox)
around 21 March

Lammas
around 1 August

Beltane
around 1 May

Litha
(Summer Solstice)
around 21 June

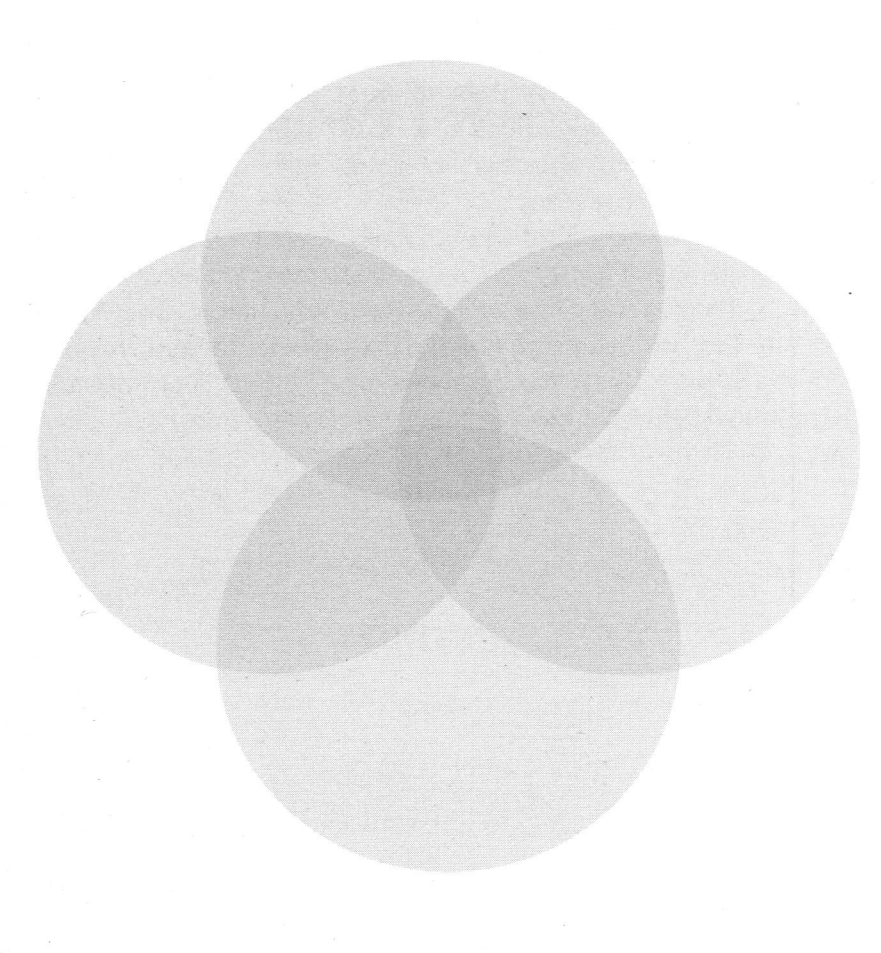

CHAPTER 5

SPRING

Spring brings a wonderful sense of new beginnings and promise. Who doesn't get excited by the new sights and sounds of spring? We feel ready to return to a more energetic way of going about things, in time with those first, reliable stirrings of nature.

We have sat with the darkest days of winter and now feel ready to invite something a little bit magical into our everyday. Whether that's embarking on a new adventure or bringing about some positive changes, we are transformed by the fresh spring air.

OSTARA (SPRING EQUINOX)

In the Wheel of the Year, Ostara is the spring equinox, which marks the first day of spring.

The name comes from Eostre, a goddess of Germanic origin, and over time this pagan date became known as Easter with the Christianization of many seasonal turning points. Even though we don't know too much about this goddess, Eostre is usually associated with fertility, dawn and rebirth.

The spring equinox certainly carries an energy of renewal. The light has returned and the earth is getting warmer, so this is a potent time to take on new challenges and do the things you may have been putting off or put to bed over winter.

If you enjoy astrology, the zodiac sign of Aries enters our space at the time of the equinox. It carries a get-the-party-started energy with its courageous and taking-charge qualities.

It's good to remember that the equinox also represents balance, as night and day are now roughly of equal length. So, it's important to unfold slowly from the sleepier days of winter. You might burn out too quickly by the time Beltane comes along if not! Take a good stretch and a big yawn, and remember to warm up those limbs after the nesting months of winter.

Even though spring is a great time to sow seeds of positivity for the weeks ahead, and become more sociable with the outside world, this time of year can cause anxiety for some folk, who feel the need to make progress but feel overwhelmed at the idea of moving out of the winter comfort zone. It's important that we feel more secure about taking a few risks before we make those all-important spring intentions of growth.

If you can't wait to make some waves, feel free to move on to the spring intentions on page 48. If you're struggling with a fear of failure, or perhaps feel anxious about taking on a new project, this practice is for you:

 ## Step out of your comfort zone

We're geared up to want the familiarity and snugness of our comfort zones, often unconsciously creating them in all corners of our lives. It's little wonder that predictability can feel like the ideal state when life is full of so many curve balls and stressful times. Trying a new plan, or adventure, might add an unwanted layer of potential embarrassment or anxiety into the mix.

But as seasons tenderly shift and change, we need to as well. Holding ourselves back may mean missed opportunities. So what can we do about it?

This practice is an NLP (Neuro-Linguistic Programming) technique I use with clients to give them a positive boost. It is a handy tool to use when anxious thoughts about change pop up.

1. Close your eyes and remember a time in your life when something great came out of trying something new. It doesn't matter what it was or when it happened; it can even be a childhood memory.
2. Bring that experience to the fore in your mind and associate any sounds, sights, smells or tastes with that time. For example, was there a song you listened to when you tried that new thing? Was there a particular smell, like a flower, cut grass or baked food that reminds you of that time? Make that experience as vivid as you can in your mind's eye.
3. Add in some emotion now. How did it feel to try something new? What good things came from the experience? What did you appreciate and what did you learn?
4. With one hand, touch your thumb and forefinger together, while you "play the movie" of your memory in your mind. This helps you to root into what you felt, saw and heard.
5. Now, think of a word that makes you feel really good about challenging yourself, such as "growth", "brave" or anything that feels right for you.
6. Open your eyes when you are ready. In the future, when you need a boost to try something new, or go about things differently, simply press together the same thumb and forefinger, saying your special word in your mind or out loud.

Set new goals

Living in flow with the seasons means we're continually expanding and letting go. The spring equinox gives us the perfect chance to take stock of our needs, set some intentions and plan some short-term and long-term goals. In this practice, we start with some groundwork. You might like to use a journal for this, or simply sit quietly to think. Ask yourself:

1. What goal would you like to achieve, this season, or in the future? Try to be as specific as possible. This can be anything such as driving somewhere new, starting a new business ...
2. Next, think about why this goal is important to you.
3. Next, think what skills and beliefs you will need to bring this goal to fruition. Getting what you want is great, but what is (usually) satisfying is the process involved in reaching that goal.
4. Finally, imagine or jot down how it will feel to accomplish this goal and what you will solve by achieving that goal.

PLANT INTENTIONS

Now we've got our goal/s straight in our heads, let's bring in a sprinkle of magic. In alignment with the Wheel of the Year and celebrating Ostara, we can work with the symbolism of fertility, abundance and life-force energy to ritualize these spring intentions, giving your goals an extra bit of moxie.

You will need:
- pan
- egg (or, if you prefer, find a beautiful round pebble)
- pens
- wildflower seeds

1. If using an egg, cook the egg in boiling water for about 10 minutes, until hard boiled. Leave to cool.
2. Decorate your egg (or pebble) with symbols, words and images that represent the goal/s you have for yourself.
3. When you've finished doing this, crack the egg and remove the shell.
4. Next, find somewhere in nature that you can bury the shell in the soil, expressing your gratitude for the earth. If you like, you can eat the egg, as a symbol of nurturing both yourself and nature.
5. Sprinkle your seeds into the soil and nourish them with water. As you do so, say out loud your goal/s and visualize your intention coming to fruition.
6. Finish by saying the mantra:

"As the season changes, I open myself up to exciting challenges for the greater good and hold space for new beginnings."

 Kitchen witchen

One easy way to live in alignment with the seasons is to eat seasonal foods. These are harvested at their peak, which means you're eating them when they are at their most nutritious and delicious. It's also a great way to reduce your carbon footprint as you're not buying food that's been imported from all over the world. Some great foods to eat during spring are:

- asparagus
- spinach
- spring cabbages
- spring onions/scallions
- purple sprouting broccoli
- radishes
- lettuces
- new potatoes
- peas
- raspberries
- rhubarb

SPRING SALAD

This is a delicious spring salad with fresh, seasonal vegetables and vibrant colours. It's packed with polyphenol-rich foods – colourful fruits, vegetables, legumes and herbs. Research suggests eating foods containing polyphenols and antioxidants can lower blood sugar levels, lower the risk of heart disease and boost cognitive performance. A delicious way to increase your fibre intake and help balance your hormones.

Choose whatever quantities you like, depending on what you have. Simply mix:

- asparagus (this can be blanched, cooked or raw)
- radishes
- spinach
- red leaf lettuce
- spring onions/scallions
- chickpeas/garbanzo beans (roasted is nice here)
- peas (these can be thawed frozen peas or fresh)
- feta or other crumbly cheese
- mint
- basil
- extra virgin olive or cold-pressed rapeseed oil
- white wine vinegar
- freshly ground black pepper and sea salt

And serve!

BELTANE

As spring picks up the pace and the wheel turns, we can celebrate Beltane, Beltine or Beltaine, which is halfway between the spring equinox and summer solstice. Beltane is all about love, sexuality, prosperity, radiance, potential and creativity.

Beltane is often discussed as being one of the four-quarter fire festivals in the Celtic year. What is more likely is that Beltane and Samhain (autumn) divided the year into two halves, with Beltane being the time of the "masculine" and Samhain representing the "feminine". The exact history may be unknown, but what we can ritualize is the earth's natural heat and growth.

Fertility, abundance and richness represent Beltane, as right now, the earth's energy is powerful and our natural surroundings are flourishing. Dancing around a maypole, making flower crowns, making a wish by a hawthorn tree or enjoying bonfire parties with friends are some traditional ways to celebrate Beltane.

For me, Beltane has a sexy energy. As life is full to bursting, it's a celebration of our sensuality and our senses. The burning energies of Beltane infuse our bodies with its powerful wild forces, compelling us feel more energized and sexual. From simmer pots to sex/tantric rituals, there are many ways to spice things up a little in tune with the burning energies of Beltane. What kind of things make you feel energized?

Many witchy folk like to look to the world of mythology to deepen the occasion. Perhaps getting to know Freya, the Norse goddess of love, may spark your creative fire. Or is it the naughty spirits or faeries who can supposedly cross between the spirit and physical world when the veil is thin? Or the deity, Belenus, with his protective powers? However you choose to deepen your seasonal practices, it's your intention that will always be most valuable.

CREATE A SIMMER POT

Fill a medium-sized saucepan just over halfway with tap water or water from a natural source, such as a river or the sea. You can also use moon water (see pages 105–6). Allow the water to simmer but not to boil. Stir in fresh or dried seasonal herbs and flowers. Lavender, thyme, rose petals and sliced lemon work beautifully at Beltane. If you want to attract something into your life, stir clockwise. If you want to let go of something, stir counter-clockwise. You can simmer the water for an hour or two, enjoying the aroma filling your home. When nearly all the water has evaporated, turn off the heat. You can dispose of your simmer pot leftovers in the compost bin or make an offering to a Beltane goddess of your choice by pouring it back into the earth.

Beltane writing prompt: passion

Beltane brings an appraisal of your spring intentions. What would you like to move forward with this peak of spring energies? Journalling your ideas stokes the fire of self-development. Some questions you may like to ask yourself are:

- What experiences would you like to have and what experiences are you already grateful for?
- How are you treating yourself as spring expands? What can you do to love yourself a little harder?
- How are you on track to bring your goals to fruition?
- Is there anything that prevents your passions from growing?
- How do you celebrate the pleasures of living?
- What fuels your spirit?

Beltane incantation

Incantations are little magic formulas of language. A bit like chanting, incantations can be used to empower your self-growth and solidify your intentions. I've included a witchy incantation for each of the seasons, but you're welcome to write your own. When you say your incantation, feel free to decorate a sacred space in your home with some fresh flowers or go for a Beltane walk to soak in the rising heat of late spring.

With winter's cocoon burning away,
The sun's strength finally has its say.
As the fire infuses our highest vision,
Our potential and creativity call for precision.
Passions build and spring spells unfold,
Helping us separate the new from the old.
Not a celebration of complete certainty,
Simply, a red-hot reminder to act purposely.
A Beltane promise of expression and worth,
As radiant love is invited to birth.

Tending to our personal growth gives us the power to transform old habits and bring clarity to our intentions. Our minds, bodies and souls are stirring once more with the earth's rising energy, bringing excitement and hope. Saying yes to this newness adds juice to our dreams as the days extend and the earth becomes warmer. This challenges us to be courageous, but grounded, as we learn to nurture our strengths and engage with the outside world more passionately and creatively. When summer has its way, we'll be ready to bloom.

CHAPTER 6

SUMMER

Summer has finally arrived. With clear, blue skies and the sound of nature turned up to its full volume, many of us feel our best during the summer months. It's a time to get together with others, enjoy evenings outside and celebrate everything life has to offer. Both people and nature are at their energetic peak so we can capitalize on these expansive energies by going that extra mile.

Fun, laughter, pleasure, playfulness, high energy and passion projects are the name of the game. However, if you feel overwhelmed with goals, or feeling burnt-out, you may have a feeling of impending doom when summer taps at the door.

To help us live in alignment with the year, let's get to know what the summer equinox symbolizes, clear away any unwanted blocks, and consciously maximize the season.

LITHA (SUMMER SOLSTICE)

Litha is the summer solstice in the Wheel of the Year, which marks the first day of summer. Litha is the Anglo-Saxon word for June, while solstice means "sun standing still" in Latin. The sun has reached its highest point in the sky, and from now on the sun will set earlier each night until the winter solstice.

SACRED PLACES

Many ancient sacred sites were established to monitor the cycles of the sun. If possible, I recommend making a pilgrimage to a place you feel drawn to. Avebury Henge, Glastonbury Tor, Stonehenge, Clava Cairns, Pentre Ifan, Ffynone Waterfall, Hill of Tara, the Fairy Pools on the Isle of Skye and The Storr have been my favourite places to visit these past few years. Quitting the very efficient world for a short while helps crystalize our cyclical practice and feel connected to the true meaning of life. What pockets of power do you feel the pull to explore? By visiting sacred lands, we're reminded that we belong. Whether it's the lands of your people or a place you have an affinity with, you're connecting to the web of the life where everything and everyone is connected.

There are many deities associated with the power of the sun. In neo-pagan traditions, Midsummer tells the story of The Oak King, who is the ruler of summer, and The Holly King, who is the ruler of winter, confronting each other in battle to fight for the crown. The Gaelic word for oak is "duir", meaning doorway. The solstice represents crossing a threshold or making an entrance into "the next". It's this metaphorical doorway that serves as a great reminder to check in on what we've been working toward, take accountability for our goals, celebrate the achievements we've made since the spring equinox (no matter how big or small), and reassess any previous intentions. This doesn't have to look anything more than a "Huh, this hasn't worked so well, how might I go about this instead?" or, "This is such a great step toward me bringing this goal to life!"

The summer solstice has a go-big-or-go-home kinda feel, so showing up can feel great here, but that doesn't mean that you need to rush into anything too serious or regimented. It's still very much a time of letting your hair down and having some fun.

The nurturing zodiac sign of Cancer marks the time of the summer solstice, which can help you to take stock of your year and understand how you feel about things. This sign will help you deepen your self-care practices and magnetize any dreams, in a grounded and loving way.

Sometimes, the "peak" energy at this time of year can bring about feelings of anxiety. This summer feeling of needing to get stuff done and show up to the world can trigger a fear of failure, resulting in self-sabotage behaviour for some of us. Recognizing when such patterns tend to come to the fore, and having some actionable tips ready for when they do, can help us understand and enhance our cyclical living experience. We will explore this in our next practice.

 Attachment and self-esteem

For us to say yes to the world and maximize our potential, we may need to work on any self-limiting beliefs that undercut progress and bring goals to fruition. Often, self-sabotaging patterns can be rooted in childhood and the type of attachment style we experienced growing up.

The three main Westernized attachment styles are: secure, anxious and avoidant. They're impacted by how attention, love and care were shown and modelled to us growing up. Our type of attachment affects the relationships we have with others and with ourselves.

A secure attachment is usually due to a reassuring and responsive relationship with the caregiver, resulting in a healthy communication style and good self-esteem. An avoidant attachment can result in pushing others away as a result of the caregiver being preoccupied or downplaying the child's emotions. An anxious attachment refers to the persistent need for validation experienced as a result of unpredictable caregiving.

If caregivers don't relate to us in a way that feeds our self-esteem, we may behave in ways that confirm any underlying (and untrue) beliefs about not being good enough in our adult lives. When this negative behaviour inevitably sabotages the goal or idea, it can result in a "self-fulfilling prophecy" e.g. "I knew I wasn't up to the job".

Some examples of self-sabotaging behaviour include putting off a task due to a fear of failure, due to perfectionist or controlling tendencies, or in an attempt to hide emotional trauma to avoid getting hurt. It can affect many areas of life, such as work, relationships, finances and health.

NEURODIVERSITY

Neurotypical social skills are seen as the "correct" way to socialize, so some neurodivergent people find the sociability of summer especially difficult. If you are struggling with this season or find yourself social masking, talking to a professional can be a positive first step toward finding out what support is available to you. This does not mean that you need to change, or be "fixed" in any way, and you will find your own ways to embrace this season.

Scrap self-sabotage

This practice is designed to help you let go of self-sabotaging thoughts, whatever their origins. By asking yourself these questions, you can help yourself to stay focused on making small steps to resolve any negative beliefs.

You will need:
- pen
- paper or a journal

1. Firstly, write down some of the ways you undermine yourself. Recognizing patterns and having them there in plain view is sometimes half the battle.
2. Next, take a look at your values. These can be anything you hold dear to your heart, such as integrity, gratitude, perseverance, respect and kindness. See them as your guiding light in life.
3. Now, ask yourself: does my behaviour match up with my values? If they don't, what's preventing me from going about my life in a way that lines up with these values?
4. Now ask when and where did you learn to doubt yourself? Write it all down.
5. Next, think about what changes you would like to see in your behaviour and actions. How do you feel when you make progress?
6. Now, think about what would help you feel worthy of success. Some examples I've used with clients include:

   - Celebrate your small "wins". Instead of just thinking of the final "result", it's better to take little steps toward what you want and be generous with yourself when you do make any progress forward.

2. When you finish writing, light the candle and gaze into the glow. As you do so, say your words of appreciation out loud. The flickering flame melts away your worries and opens you up to abundance and power.
3. When you've finished, blow out the candle. Now fold up your piece of paper, and pop it under your pillow. Sleep on it that night.
4. On each of the 11 nights, perform the same ritual, adding another piece of paper with fresh self-appreciation, to your collection underneath your pillow.
5. At the end of the 11th day, re-read all the amazing ways you actively appreciated caring for yourself. Congratulate yourself for investing time in yourself to feel good.

You can carry on with daily words of self-appreciation after the ritual has ended for as long as you wish.

 Kitchen witchen

What better way to nurture yourself than to create a delicious and healthy meal or snack. You are worthy of the thought and effort that goes into buying and putting together seasonal food. Here are some great foods to enjoy during the summer months:

- beetroot/beets
- strawberries
- raspberries
- cherries
- cucumber
- salad leaves/greens
- green beans

- courgettes/zucchini
- summer squashes
- carrots
- tomatoes
- fennel

SUMMER BERRY ICE-CREAM

This recipe uses colourful, seasonal fruit mixed with fermented yoghurt and seeds to diversify and support your gut health. You can have it for breakfast, as a snack or as a dessert. If using fresh fruit, you will need to freeze the berries first, before making this delicious ice-cream.

If you live somewhere you can pick wild berries, such as blackberries, it's lovely to go on a mindful summer walk to connect with the season and forage goodies for snacks.

You will need:
- 150g/5oz frozen raspberries, strawberries, blueberries and/or blackberries
- 150g/5oz kefir yogurt
- a drizzle of raw honey
- 1 tbsp chia seeds

1. Put all the ingredients into a food processor and whizz until it comes together into an ice-cream texture. Serve!

LAMMAS

As summer moves forward so does the Wheel of the Year, and we are reminded that the last few weeks of the season are upon us. Lammas, or Lughnasadh, celebrates the final fullness of the season before the darker days of autumn invite us back home for some slower self-care. This is when the first loaves are baked and shared from the first harvest, representing a time of gratitude and abundance.

Lammas celebrates the sun god Lugh's foster Mother Tailtiu, the last queen of the Fir Bolg, who died of exhaustion trying to clear a large area of woodland for planting so her people could prosper. There are many variations of the story and conflicting opinions as to the origin of the myth, but a key theme throughout is a time of change, regeneration and paving the way for new energy to enter the year.

Many women will resonate with this tale of Tailtiu and the art of sacrifice. We can see that women give so much of themselves to enable, or fit in with, the expectations and needs of others. It's also a reminder that sometimes we need to make difficult choices to bring what matters to fruition, and we shouldn't always do what is considered "easy". There can be contradiction within this, and I love the idea of two opposites being true at the same time. I see Lammas as a time to move forward fearlessly, but not to the detriment of your authenticity or value.

 Lammas writing prompt: fulfilment

Lammas acts as a good reminder to take care of anything in your life that you've been meaning to bring to fulfilment. Some Lammas questions to ask yourself are:

- What needs some extra attention?
- Is there anything you would like to make a final push on?
- Where are you stopping yourself from being of service to yourself, and the world around you?
- Who are you giving too much of your time to?
- Are you showing yourself daily recognition of raising your self-worth?
- What talents are you not announcing to the world?

CELEBRATE WITH CREATIVITY

This festival can get your "make-the-most-of-it" creative juices flowing. Feel free to use this time to make a corn dolly, a traditional symbol of good luck. To make a dolly, gather stalks of grasses, wheat and barley and plait together. Or, if you're good with dough, bake some bread to symbolize the fruits of your labour coming to completion. I also like to decorate my altar or kitchen with seasonal yellow flowers, such as calendula or sunflowers, to symbolize the abundant and empowering energy of this sabbat.

 ## Lammas incantation

This late-summer incantation is to help you to review the year so far and summon yourself into action, if required. You can perform it outside, or in a sacred area of your home.

At Ostara, we planted seeds of desire,
With Beltane, we stirred the inward fire.
Through summer we watched our dreams grow,
As we learned the trust needed to be in flow.
Today, I am open to the abundance of all to be,
Showing gratitude for every gift and lesson to see.
I reap the harvest of my earthly goals,
Learning to relinquish what I cannot control.
With Lammas's last burst of changing power,
I embody effort and expansion at summer's final hour.

Summer self-confidence and positivity allow us to harvest the possibilities of the months gone by and stay aligned with the natural opportunities of the season. Abundance is everywhere, compelling us to celebrate our wins and feel truly alive in each moment. Any losses can provide moments of reflection and transform into deeper personal insights as we shift into the slower months ahead. I can already feel autumn peeking its head around the corner ...

CHAPTER 7

AUTUMN

With pumpkin-spiced lattes and days pulsating with autumnal magic, it's time for the season of the witch. We can reap the gains of our year so far by enjoying long walks showered in vibrant colours and cozy nights indoors.

As nature begins to descend with falling leaves, we too hear the call to turn inward. In this season, gentle reflection, shedding old ways and pulling back from anything that doesn't nourish us are this season's strengths. If you're a parent, having your kids back to school can mean more time for self-care.

Simply by sitting with ourselves, we can relax into the natural vibrations of life and listen to our intuitive senses more easily. We sometimes need to be quieter to understand what is trying to surface within us. Getting to know all our nooks and crannies can bring about a deeper sense of authenticity.

MABON (AUTUMN EQUINOX)

The autumnal equinox marks the beginning of autumn and the end of summer. Traditionally, communities would get together to celebrate the abundance of their conscientiously nurtured crops and celebrate the harvest period. The equinox is a time to be grateful for the cycle of growth, harvest and endings, while understanding the natural impermanence of life.

The son of Earth Mother Goddess, Mabon, was a hero, stolen as a baby and imprisoned in the underworld. He makes a famous appearance in the oldest Arthurian tale, Culhwch and Olwen. Mabon helps Culhwch with his series of 40 impossible tasks to win over the woman he loves.

In Wiccan communities, there are conflicting views on whether to call the autumnal equinox Mabon. You may, instead, want to bring the goddesses and deities that you feel drawn to into your space as the season shifts. I like to focus on the powerful Morrigan, who symbolizes many things, including the cycle of life and death, and is the keeper of prophecy. Morrigan is associated with ravens, war, intuition, protection and shapeshifting. It's a beautiful practice to approach stories and myths from the past with respect and humility.

The equinox is a time of equal light and dark, turning away from the high energy of summer to a more inward space of harmony and balance. Auspiciously, the zodiac sign of Libra, symbolized by a set of scales, coincides with Mabon. And with our ongoing urge to be consistently productive, Libra can help us look at life with a bit more understanding and evenness.

As nature slows down, we are reassured that it's OK to do the same. Drawing back with the longer nights allows us to let go of what no longer serves us. When we make an autumnal intention

Both creative solutions and intuition are often born when we allow a dip in energy. We can savour what's to be uncovered in our hearts and souls now that "the fields" have been cleared.

to tread more slowly, we give ourselves the chance to listen more attentively to the messages of our inner world.

But, what about if you feel held captive by your commitments, so slowing down doesn't feel like a choice? Or perhaps there is space to take it down a notch, but your self-worth feels enmeshed with getting things done. Then, autumn's call to be present in the here and now can feel challenging, agonizing or impossible. The answer: we need to stop overextending. Not so easy, I know. The way to do this is to create realistic expectations of ourselves. We need boundaries in every season, but saying no is particularly crucial during the autumn and winter months of the year. Being boundaried, especially when it comes to the needs of others, is our first autumn practice.

 ## Setting boundaries

Autumn is the season to be more considered and listen to your inner needs. And this will absolutely involve saying no. What's your immediate reaction here? Setting boundaries really is an act of self-love. If we carry on saying yes to the world now summer has passed, we reduce precious time for space and meaningful growth.

1. **Reflect:** Do you struggle to say no to things? Why? Could it be ... not being liked, harming a relationship, disappointing someone, wanting to gain approval or something else? Do you like being the agony aunt, perhaps? Curiosity is your great ally when it comes to self-healing, so compassionately wonder about your reasons.
2. **Don't over-explain:** We can feel bad for saying no, so our words end up running away with themselves. For example,

if you want to say no to a social event, practice using fewer words, such as, "That sounds lovely, but I'm going to have a quiet weekend". It may feel a bit weird at first, but the more you do it, the more empowered you'll feel.

3. **Manage commitments:** If you feel over-stretched at work, or elsewhere, try saying, "I am happy to take this on, but I will need some help when it comes to prioritizing tasks of lesser importance". Keep it simple, straightforward and from a good place.

4. **Circle of control:** Others may not like it when you say no. One thing we can never control in life is how others feel. If they react negatively, you will need to stand up for yourself by saying, "I don't like the way you're speaking to me". However, more often than not, it's the internal worry that you *may* have let them down in some way. They might be just fine! Spending time worrying about what others think will take up the extra seasonal space that you're trying to carve out for yourself. So, what you *can* control is saying no and how you present the boundaries. You can't control how others may feel. That is the naked truth of it.

MAKING A HARVEST WREATH

As a way to ritualize "being boundaried", you could make an equinox wreath from wheat and anything you can mindfully forage from outside. Hang it on or above your door to symbolically create a boundary around your home and evoke protection against anything unwanted. It also can remind you of the cyclical nature of life, while bringing a lovely autumnal aesthetic into your home.

Setting boundaries is an ongoing part of your self-care routine that will take shape and change as your needs evolve. Please don't beat yourself up for "failing" at something you couldn't fit into your life. We can't do everything!

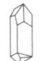 ## Being authentic

As we travel through our self-care journey, we may become increasingly aware of how other people's expectations have framed our behaviour and actions. Setting boundaries provides us with spaciousness. When we have this, we can flow more easily with our own values, instead of what others always need.

Authenticity, most simply, is what is important to you, and working out how you can act according to this.

With this in mind, let's now take time to work on letting go of some of the things that aren't authentic to your values and purpose.

 ## Living your values ritual

In this practice, we are going to look at your values, continuing from our summer practice on page 59. Values are your driving force or beacon of light that help you live with meaning; it's the parts of yourself that really matter to you. Increasing your awareness when it comes to your fulfilment will help you live authentically.

You will need:
- paper or a journal
- pen

1. Make a list of your top values, or return to the list you started in summer (see page 59). Some examples are: creativity, determination, balance, optimism, boldness, community, fairness and fun.
2. Reflect on what these values teach you and how they show up in your life.
3. Now, think about when you are most aligned with these values. How do you feel when you're able to live out and express your values?
4. Next, think about when you're *not* able to follow your values. When does life push you away from and prevent you from keeping to your values? Look at the gap between how you feel or behave in this setting and where you want to be. How can you move away from environments that aren't fulfilling?
5. Consider what actions you can bring into your life to be in alignment with your authenticity. For example, if you chose:

   - **Creativity:** You could start a side hustle that expresses this part of you or ask your boss for more creative tasks in the workplace.
   - **Community:** You could volunteer for a charity or arrange a night out.
   - **Boldness:** Look at ways you can use your boundaries and speak up for yourself.
   - **Balance:** Invite more micro-pockets of rest into your day, such as a three-minute meditation every morning.

6. Come back to your list as often as possible and look at ways that you can be more in alignment with your values. The more you do this, the easier it becomes, until flowing with your authenticity seems natural.

A NOTE ON VALUES

Re-assessing values is not always a straightforward process. Some mental health conditions may make it difficult for a person to identify and trust their values. Certain personality disorders (while understanding some diagnosed people find this term stigmatizing) may make it hard for an individual to understand themselves in the way outlined on the previous page. Some neurodivergent individuals may find that their authentic self is not "accepted" by society, so living according to one's true self is difficult. People living in abusive relationships may be required to hide their authentic selves due to survival. Please always seek professional help if you're struggling with any of these issues mentioned.

Seasonal stress

When we push against the natural rhythms of the slower months, we can increase our cortisol levels and feel more stressed. When our cortisol increases, our progesterone levels can decrease. This can cause menstrual irregularities, mood changes and sleep difficulties. Unfortunately, some of us have difficulty producing enough progesterone (we get very hormone-specific in Chapter 13) due to high levels of cortisol. The trap of seasonal stress is easy to fall into when we're faced with the incompatible needs of the outside world. Not only are we more likely to feel run down in the autumn months, but we're also contending with the decline in sunlight and the build-up to seasonal celebrations, such as Christmas. In a nutshell, we're expected to keep up the pace despite nature's call to slow down. Self-care, in all its forms, can help balance caring for your needs and meeting the ongoing demands of the outside world. If you feel stressed during this time, self-care needs to be a priority. You may like to try the recipe that follows as a lovely way to nurture your body and reduce cortisol.

 Kitchen witchen

We've nourished our minds and souls, and now we need to care for our bodies. This is the season of the kitchen witch – a pagan Thanksgiving, if you like. Many witchy folks like to gather their garden harvest and practise meditative cooking, using ingredients that are representative of things they want to bring into their life, or let go of.

Autumn presents an opportunity to cook and eat foods that warm you from the inside. Some autumn foods in season are:

- apples
- pears
- beetroot/beets
- broccoli
- carrots
- cauliflower
- celery
- kale
- leeks
- onions
- potatoes
- spinach
- squashes

SWEET POTATO HUMMUS

Let's make a hearty, autumnal dip that you can add to a toasted seeded bagel for lunch or serve as a delicious after-work (or after-school) snack, with fresh vegetable sticks. As well as being delicious, sweet potatoes are good for gut bacteria and boost our immunity. They can also help us to make progesterone by reducing cortisol (see page 177).

You will need:
- 1 sweet potato
- a good glug of extra virgin olive oil
- 240g/8oz chickpeas/garbanzo beans, drained, or 1 can of cooked chickpeas
- 3 tablespoons tahini
- 2 garlic cloves, crushed
- ½ teaspoon cumin
- juice of 1 lemon
- Celtic or pink Himalayan salt, to season

1. Roast the sweet potato in the oven at 220°C/400°F/ gas 7 for about 1 hour, until tender. When cool, peel and mash.
2. Put all the ingredients into a food processor and blend. Add a little salt, to season. Serve or store in an airtight container in the fridge for up to four days.

SAMHAIN

All of a sudden, the clocks turn back and Halloween is (quite literally) ringing the doorbell. Samhain is considered the most important of the four quarter fire festivals, marking the final harvest and the end of summer. At Samhain, it's thought that winter fires were lit, animals were sacrificed and ancestors were celebrated. The veil between the material and the underworld was said to be thin, meaning spirits could return to earth on this day. People would dress up and wear masks in an attempt to dupe any potential spirits that may cause harm. With the Christianization of many celebrations, Samhain became All Saints' Day or All Hallows, eventually becoming Halloween.

CELTIC SPIRITUALITY

"Celtic" is sometimes used to describe what would have been a hugely varied experience, including diverse geographical areas, communities, contrasting beliefs, practices and ways of working with nature. The Samhain festival, and its modern manifestation as Halloween, is a way to enter into the rituals of the past. The many practices and ways of the past have been distorted or relayed incorrectly under the buzz term of Celtic spirituality, which really, covers so many things. Studying the original history surrounding your ancestors can help your journey of spirituality and the way you connect to the land.

As the Wheel of the Year turns and we find ourselves knee-deep in autumnal magic, we are urged to acknowledge our shadow selves. Samhain is a time of endings, encouraging us to go deeper into the darkness so that we can pave space for transformation.

It's much more comfortable (and sometimes completely necessary) to stay put in life, covering up or avoiding the parts of ourselves we don't like. But if we don't take time to get to know ourselves fully, old triggers and unhelpful behaviours will never die off.

 ## Shadow work

This season is the ideal time to explore shadow work. This is simply taking time to reflect on any limiting beliefs you might carry, to improve self-awareness and self-acceptance. You can explore the relationship you have with yourself, and with others. This can sometimes involve wondering about your childhood experiences and how you were brought up.

Sitting with, and accepting, the shadow sides of yourself will mean you need to put aside any feelings of shame. Your shadow side is simply longing for a little tenderness and acceptance, and so curiosity is all you need here. In our next practice, we will explore shadow work with some questions around this season.

 ## Samhain writing prompt: shadow work

Let's get all kinds of curious about the less "appetizing" parts of you with some Samhain journaling. Please only do shadow work if you feel it is right for your circumstances.

You will need:
- paper or a journal
- pen

1. What makes you feel at peace?
2. What makes you feel uneasy?
3. What sort of person do you attract into your space?
4. Which relationship patterns do you tend to repeat?
5. What are, or were, your caregiver's values? Are your personal values the same or different?
6. What versions of yourself do you hide from others or hope that no one sees?
7. What do people get wrong about you?
8. What do you wish others knew about you?
9. When do you feel like you don't match up?
10. What are your secret regrets?
11. What needs to change to feel more self-accepting ? And how would that feel?

There's not much to "do" following this practice. Deeply acknowledging the process, in the same way that nature doesn't force the timings of things, shows us that we don't need to "modify" ourselves to be OK. That doesn't mean to say we can't strive or embrace change when the time is right – nature does both of these things to perfection. It simply means that when we walk through Samhain's gateway, we are reminded that there is a time for everything. This season is a restful space to fully sit with ourselves as the intuitive stillness of winter approaches.

Samhain incantation

With a sprinkle of magic, we can celebrate Samhain with a few words to consolidate the importance of turning inward and show an appreciation of the void. This would be lovely to do outside as the sun is setting, or in a sacred area of your home.

> *At Mabon, I allowed sensitivity and intuition,*
> *Showing gratitude for dreams coming to fruition.*
> *As the void descends and nights stretch longer,*
> *The howl of my innermost self becomes stronger.*
> *With Samhain, I am called to gaze into the dark,*
> *Unafraid to listen, I allow true potential to spark.*
> *Honouring my ancestors, I celebrate both life and death,*
> *As the season takes its final fading breaths.*
> *Now I turn inwards, gathering nutrients to store,*
> *Only then, can new possibilities rise once more.*

Taking time to connect with ourselves and the natural world feels empowering in autumn. When we choose to move with the seasons and go against the modern-day set-up of consistency, we embody the strengths of self-respect and surrender. "Holding onto" only holds us back from change. And change is just as much about shedding as it is about achieving. Have faith in the gifts of each season as we move into the quietest months ... I promise winter is super-special when you let it be so.

CHAPTER 8

WINTER

Yes please, winter duvet!

As nature sinks into stillness, we are supposed to dial it down and preserve our energy for the lighter days ahead. It's a season to go within, which is why the usual, excessive festivities at this time of year can go against our natural need for quiet.

Despite the slower, cozy appeal of winter, women can feel more pressured and stressed than ever during this season. How else can we manage the ongoing work, family and life commitments otherwise? We might feel the need to cut corners and get things ticked off as quickly as possible to keep up the pace.

I'm not suggesting you ghost everyone and live alone in the woods. But proper self-care must be prioritized. Coping strategies, good sleep and a touch of selfishness are essential to reducing winter seasonal stress (see page 216).

Let's get into the strengths of this season and give ourselves permission to rest a little deeper.

YULE (WINTER SOLSTICE)

On the shortest day of the year, the winter solstice marks the beginning of winter and the return of the light. It's the longest night and the shortest day of the year. The winter solstice is a lovely time of reflection, hibernation and spending time with loved ones. It's the season to keep yourself warm with soothing hot drinks, fluffy blankets and cozy socks.

Leaning into the mystical side of things, we can celebrate this beautiful duality by honouring the winter goddess, Cailleach. She is a veiled Crone (see Chapter 4) who represents death, protection and transformation.

It's thought that the modern-day pagan festival of Yule has roots in Norse or Germanic traditions. Early pagan groups celebrated what was then Jól with large feasts and animal sacrifices. As with many festivals, it's difficult to know the exact history, but it's thought that a Yule log was burnt in the fireplace to represent darkness and symbolize the return of the light.

What does winter look like for you where you live? I'm aware that it's not always the snowy rolling hills captured on screen. For those of us with little sunlight, this season can feel like a time to hibernate and put ourselves back together again. As nature flutters its eyes closed, we are quietly persuaded to do the same.

WINTER AND LONELINESS

When it's cold outside, we are more likely to feel lonely. Feeling lonely isn't the same as choosing to be alone. Nearly half of adults living in the UK have said they feel lonely at times, with women being more affected than men. Joining a walking group, starting a class or volunteering can be a wonderful way to combat loneliness. If this isn't possible, or feels too intimidating, going for a winter wander or listening to a funny podcast can feel easier.

Yet the noisy excess of the festive period and all its trappings is often more convincing, so we end up doing too much and burning out before the new year even begins. That said, I encourage coming together with people you love, as many past communities would have done during the Yule period, but in a way that's slower and soul-nourishing.

The pragmatic zodiac sign of Capricorn will help us keep the buzz of Christmas more grounded. Yes, this sign is motivated by achievements, but success can look like whatever you want it to. One way to capitalize on Capricorn's discipline is to get serious about the deepest self-care. I hear you – this isn't always easy. I find self-care difficult when my two burnt-out kids are off school for the festive period. The first step is to keep our winter practices realistic, and not try to do everything. The second is to abandon any harsh New Year's resolutions.

However, there is one thing I would love you to try: take a break from social media and phone use. Too much social media use (especially at night) can have a negative effect on the mind and body. The blue light of screens can decrease our melatonin production, affecting our sleep quality. Relationships may be affected due to "phubbing" (ignoring a loved one due to looking at your phone), and jealous feelings of being left out when seeing a friend's social media post at a festive event can also affect our wellbeing. It's so easy to get hooked on "doomscrolling" in the hope that it gives us a hit of something we're craving, and the dopamine high of getting likes and comments on your own posts can feel great. Social media has been designed to make us feel this very way, after all. However, winter is a time to come away from all this noise.

Digital detox

Even though we humans find moderation tricky, it's important to remind ourselves that we're in control of our phone use. Taking even one week off social media can help us connect to the real world, reduce stress, improve sleep and cope better during winter.

1. Choose a good week to come off social media. This will give you a realistic head start. Quieter for many, the week between Christmas and New Year may be an optimum time to detox.
2. Ask a friend or family members if they want to do it with you. This encourages accountability.
3. Tell your friends and family you're still around for phone calls and messages to stay feeling connected.
4. Schedule a winter catch-up or two (a winter walk and talk is great), especially if you're worried about FOMO.
5. During your detox, remind yourself of the benefits with a mantra, such as: "My worth is tied to kind words, time to be present, feeling enough and living in the flow".

ENJOY WINTER

There are so many lovely ways to enjoy this slower time. Why not try something from the list below? These activities also remind you of how in control of your time you can be, without needing to look at your phone. All of these things will make you feel good, I promise, without the unnecessary sting of comparison or envy. Scrolling is just a way to feel connected so let's create healthier ways to achieve this and heal the comparison gap. Think of this as your mini hibernation time.

- Gaze out the window with a hot drink while listening to the muted sounds of winter.
- Go for stroll along a beach, through a park or perhaps in the evening, look up at the stars with wonder. Go with a friend, if you prefer.
- Spend a while choosing an outfit that makes you feel good.
- Prepare some delicious, warming food while listening to music that you love.
- Practise meditation.
- Donate to a food bank.
- Upon waking, write down your dreams in a beautiful notebook. This is an interesting way to gain personal insight or receive intuitive messages. Dreams whisper clues about our waking lives and create awareness around what needs to be healed.
- Send a friend a card with a cute message or funny poem.

 Sleep soundly ritual

Sleep is so important in every season, but we may be prone to feeling especially lethargic if we don't have good sleep in winter. Sleep is one of the best ways to reset your body health and has the added benefit of increasing longevity. If you have experienced low mood in previous winters, focusing on sleep and not feeling the pressure to be out late every night can really help.

- Alcohol can really impact on your sleep. Ditch the evening drink as it will clutter your sleep with more frequent wakings.
- Try not to crank up the winter heating in your bedroom and keep it nice and cool.
- Keep your bedroom dark to increase melatonin levels.
- Never check emails or scroll through your phone before sleep.
- Go to bed at the same time every night to help regulate your circadian rhythm.
- Try not to press the snooze button in the morning as this can harm your cardiovascular system; it's better to get out of bed when you wake naturally.

SEASONAL AFFECTIVE DISORDER

Permitting yourself to go slower and sleep more during winter isn't the same as having seasonal affective disorder (SAD). SAD is a diagnosable depression that affects approximately one in twenty people at the same time every year, usually in winter. One of the symptoms is sleeping for longer than normal and feeling especially demotivated and sluggish during the day. Going for an early walk, as close to waking as possible, can help regulate your circadian rhythm, improve vitamin D levels and reduce symptoms of depression. Cognitive behavioural therapy and light therapy boxes can also help with SAD. If you're concerned, it's always good to speak to a professional.

Kitchen witchen

As our minds need tending to, our bodies need the same loving attention. Here are some lovely fruits and veggies to explore in the winter months:

- Brussels sprouts
- celeriac
- celery
- horseradish
- parsnips
- cabbage
- swede/rutabaga
- onions
- mushrooms
- oranges
- apples

FERMENTED FIRE CIDER

A winter non-alcoholic brew can blow the cobwebs away, boost our immune system and reduce inflammation. Fermenting foods at home, such as jars of garlic in honey, has become a popular way to combat sore throats and improve gut health. Mix up this fiery brew and take a spoonful each day for a little kick of energy.

You will need:
- 5 garlic cloves, peeled
- 1 thumb horseradish, peeled

- 1 thumb root ginger, peeled
- 1 red chilli
- 1 red or white onion, peeled
- 500ml/16fl oz raw cider vinegar
- 1 orange
- 3 tbsp honey (raw is great)
- 1 cinnamon stick

1. Chop the garlic, horseradish, ginger, onion and chilli.
2. Zest the orange. Put them all into a sterile 1 litre/35fl oz jar.
3. Pour over the cider vinegar and stir.
4. Add the honey, cinnamon stick and juice from the orange. Make sure all the ingredients are submerged.
5. Store the jar in a dark cupboard or larder to ferment for at least a week, and up to four weeks. After then, store in the fridge for up to six weeks.
6. Drink a tablespoon of the liquid each day (leaving behind the chopped ingredients).

IMBOLC

Just as winter feels like it's never going to leave, we start to see the first signs of life pushing through the landscape at Imbolc. Imbolc is a seasonal fire festival celebrating the awakening of Mother Earth. It's unknown as to how far back in history the festival of Imbolc reaches, but it's likely to have been celebrated in areas inhabited by Gaelic-speaking people.

The renewal of Imbolc in the pagan Wheel of the Year pulls us toward the idea of a shift in energy, from the darkest of days, to potential and new beginnings.

We can call upon the goddess Brigid during this time. Creating a Brigid cross with reeds, drinking chamomile tea, lighting a candle or having a wild swim are lovely ways to celebrate this potent goddess and the festival of Imbolc. In Irish mythology, Brigid was the daughter of the Dagda and potentially the Morrigan, who were members of the supernatural race, Tuatha Dé Danann. With her magical cloak, Brigid was able to heal and protect the sick. As with all goddesses (and women), she was complete with contradiction, representing many different sides of the female experience. She is associated with fertility, water, fire, serenity, childbirth, the home, weaponry and poetry.

Imbolc is a time of differences. Depending on where you live, the days are often their most chilly but we begin to stir from the hypnotic depths of winter with more light. This is a magical time to honour the winter season by allowing space for intuition and reflection while becoming gently seduced by the hopefulness of spring.

 Imbolc writing prompt: lessons

This gentle Imbolc inquiry invites you to optimize your closing winter energies. Take this time here to heal from your season's lessons and think about where you want to take things in the future.

- What are your biggest winter lessons?
- What are you dreaming of and what does this tell you?
- What are you opening up to?
- What patterns linger that need attention or care?

- What areas of your home need to be cleared or changed?
- What new buds of creativity or change are stirring within you and where would you like to take this?

 Imbolc incantation

As with each of the quarter festivals, saying an incantation can seal our healing journey and create seasonal intentions. This is best said outside or in a sacred area of your home, especially as the sun is rising.

Inviting those Yule intentions to gently extend,
Knowing the stillness of the season will soon end.
For now, it's not what we have to show,
As growth is surrendering to the slow.
Wrapped in Brigid's cloak of protection,
We're afforded space for the deepest reflection.
And by defending soft inner knowing a little longer,
Those seeds of creativity take time to grow stronger.
As spring potential feels closer to taste,
Gently unfurling at Imbolc without hustle or haste.

In winter, you don't need to "do" to be magical. The longer nights slowly seduce us into stillness, where we hand over our need to be productive for a while. Purpose is now sitting with quiet moments and letting things be. Without this darkness, new ideas and inspirations aren't able take root when the light comes back. A time of endings and beginnings, we bring our earth practices to a close as we look up to the sky to ritualize our connection with the moon.

PART THREE

LUNAR CYCLE

Hello again, lunettes.

We began our cyclical journey with the four seasons of our life cycle. Looking to nature, we expanded our self-care practices through the eyes of the earth's seasons. Now, we can stretch a little higher in the light of the moon (lunar) phases. As we explore our understanding of the lunar phases, we also return home to our closest cycle, learning to live in flow with our menstrual seasons.

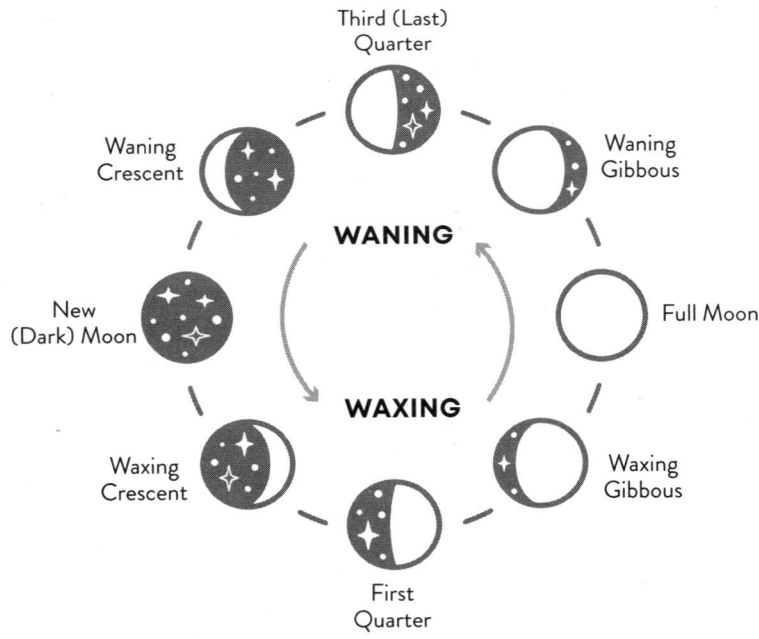

Are you someone who feels calmer at the new moon, or perhaps you find sleeping difficult at the full moon? We know the moon influences the tides, and as our bodies are 60 per cent water, we may find our internal systems naturally ebb and flow with the moon's phases on a spiritual level.

Interest about the moon's impact on a person's health can be traced back to Ancient Greece and Rome, where full moons were associated with "erratic" behaviour. It's also believed that a woman's menstrual cycle was closely linked to the moon, before the invention of electricity, when we lived more in keeping with light and dark. There has been a lot of research into our human connection to the moon – one study indicates that the full moon affects our ability to sleep at night, with results showing that participants took longer to fall asleep and experienced a reduction in deep sleep. However, some explain any connection as a self-fulfilling prophecy, in that some people might change their behaviour because they believe they're supposed to.

Although the jury is out on how the moon affects the body through the lens of current scientific research, people have been spellbound by its charm. From the early humans who observed the course of the moon as a way of timekeeping, to the ancient moon temples and ceremonial sites set up as places of worship, the moon's power is embedded in our history. And it's not just people that are affected. Certain marine species, including reef coral and some fish species, have reproductive cycles timed with the moon.

My feeling is that some people are more susceptible to the seasons of the moon than others. It might be that things come to a head for you during the full moon, while some of you may hardly feel her influence. What I'm most interested in is how we can deepen our cyclical self-development in the context of something greater than ourselves. And no matter where we are, we all gaze up to the same exceptional moon.

- Move away from all-or-nothing thinking. You are not your thoughts, so creating some distance between yourself and your thinking patterns can be a positive step forward.
- Practise mindfulness to gain perspective. There are lots of ideas for this in this book (see pages 156, 184 and 213), but simply focusing on your breathing for a few minutes, right now, is a simple way to calm the mind and focus on the moment, rather than on worries and concerns.

 ## Self-appreciation ritual

As we're working on showing up to the world with the wonderfully powerful and climactic summer energies, we first need to be OK with showing up for ourselves. This can take time and needs gentle persistence.

In numerology, the number 11 is connected to a higher source of wisdom. This ritual is to be carried out every day, for 11 consecutive days, to create consistency and symbolize the cool cosmicality of this number.

You will need:
- pen
- paper
- candle, of your choosing

1. At the end of each of the 11 days, write down three positive things that you've done, to show appreciation for yourself. This can be as simple as "I said no to that person who was asking too much from me", or "I cooked myself a delicious and nourishing dinner".

On a spiritual level, the new moon and full moon are pivotal points in cyclical living as they provide opportunities to assess self-development. It's thought that the moon has a feminine or yin energy that calls us to be in tune with our most intimate emotional state. And for this reason, I use "she" when referring to the moon. Each moon phase can be seen as a gateway to living in alignment with our truth.

The waxing and waning moons can be categorized as crescent, quarter and gibbous. I have grouped "the energies" together in honour of our need for simplicity without dismissing the nuances of each micro stage.

It's also worth noting that the moon moves between each of the 12 signs of the zodiac, falling into different signs every full and new moon. As I'm not an astrologist nor an expert on this, I have kept to the theme of the four main seasons (as I have done in each of the chapters) as a way of enhancing everyday living, but feel free to open out to more ways of working with the moon. As the moon carries a mystical energy, some of these sessions will feel "witchy". There are times for logic and times for magic, so you can feel free to dip in and out of them as it feels right to you.

Some witchy folk like to follow the Celtic Tree Calendar, which is divided by the 13 moon cycles of the year. Each of the 13 months is named after a tree, with the moon cycles being used to ascertain the best time for planting crops. It's based on (or borrowed from) the early Irish Ogham alphabet. Even though there is no evidence to believe the calendar comes from ancient times, it can still act as a way to connect with both the moon and the land because spirituality is always a deeply personal practice.

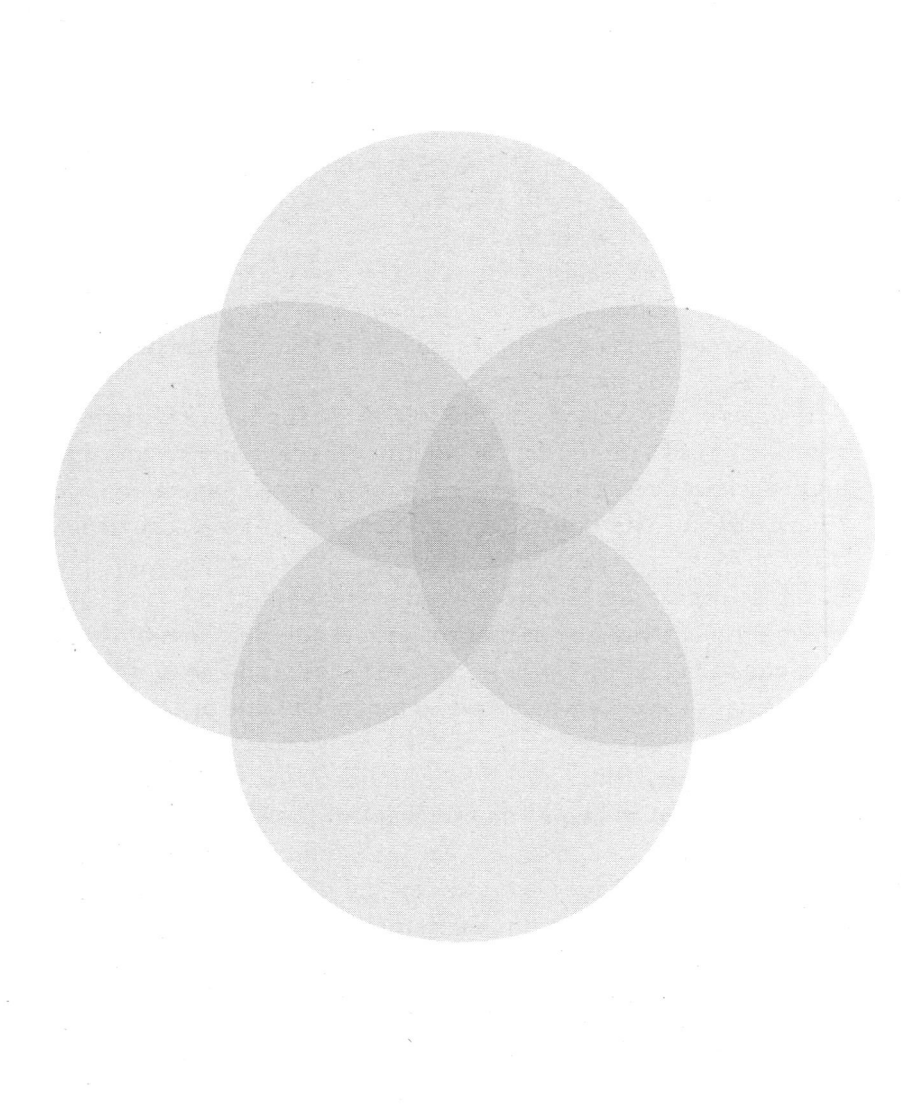

CHAPTER 9

NEW MOON

Ready to make a wish?

The new moon is a cauldron of possibility and new beginnings. At this time, the moon can't be seen – imagine she's an empty container waiting for you to set your intentions for the month ahead. The new moon has a quieter, restful energy, so this process is best done from a calm, centred place. You can do this by yourself, or gather with your coven, to sow seeds together and reap even greater success. You might like to choose to do this in an esbat.

An esbat is a coven meeting held during the full or new moon where rituals, spells and healing work happen. They are an opportunity to commune with goddesses and the divine.

PERFECTING OUR MANIFESTATIONS

In the spirit of being all wild about the moon, when we set and manifest our intentions we can make them **RAVE,** to get purpose-driven without the pressure:

- **Respectful:** It's important that your intention is respectful and for the highest good. What I mean by that is there should be an ethical or moral standard with wishes. For example, the wish should be about personal growth or a positive goal that reaches beyond the self, but never about control, harm or needing someone else to change. Ask yourself, how would my goal positively affect my life and the lives of others?

- **Achievable:** Making your intentions realistic allows them to feel attainable and increases the likelihood of them coming to fruition. This will help you create a good routine and stay consistent. For example, developing a personality trait, such as flexibility; improving an area of your wellbeing, such as sleep; or boosting abundance by creating a side business.

- **Values-led:** Choose to make your intention aligned with your values. So, if one of your top values is health, your intention could be "I eat healthy, nourishing foods". Putting the intention in the present moment and ensuring it is entirely positive makes it feel like it's already happening. Avoid a statement like, "I will avoid unhealthy food". As a hypnotherapist and NLP practitioner, I love the idea of opting for empowering language to cultivate positivity. Values-led intentions will help push you on, filling the desires with momentum to move forward.

- **Emotional:** Think about how your intention will make you feel. For example, if you're manifesting prosperity, focus on the feeling you want to attract into your life. Is it a sense of belonging, is it more time and space, is it more adventure? Get transparent about what you want and why. That doesn't mean you want to become too attached to the outcome, but just gives you more clarity.

Lunar ritual: manifestation

At the new moon, carve out some time to set your intentions and create a manifestation sigil to imbue your goals with magic.

You will need:
- paper
- pens
- matches or lighter
- fire-proof bowl

1. Make yourself comfortable and take a few deep breaths in and out through your nose.
2. When you feel settled, write down your intentions for the month ahead, remembering to make them RAVE (see page 95–6). When you're finished, read them out loud.
3. Now cross out the vowels and repeated letters in your intention. For example, if your intention was, "I invite prosperity", it would look like: NVTPRSY.
4. Next, create, or doodle, an abstract symbol based on the letters, guided by your subconscious. It doesn't matter what it looks like. When doodling on this intention, this is what I came up with, as an example.

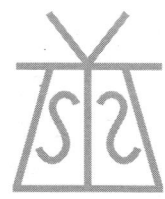

5. Close your eyes and meditate on the drawing in your mind's eye. This is where you're able to see and visualize things with the mind. Say your intention out loud as you do so.
6. Next, to charge the energy of the sigil, burn the paper.
7. Let the magic do its work!

MANIFESTATION AND PRIVILEGE

Unfortunately, there is a sombre side to manifestation. In some cases, people have given lots of money and time to "spiritual guides" claiming to help them manifest their desires, without much to show for it. There's also the issue that manifestation ignores socio-economic reality. If we look at the wheel of privilege, which takes into consideration race, gender, education, sexuality, abilities and wealth, we are more likely to achieve our goals based on how close we are to the centre of power. I believe we can aspire to evolve while being aware of the inherent privilege we may be carrying. We can dream while having a profound compassion for those in less-privileged positions. And we can strive for personal fulfilment while advocating for the rights of others.

Under the darkness of the moon, we sink into the potential of new starts. In this celestial reset, we're tuned into the whispers of our hearts, and it's from this attentive listening that we create intentions that count. With the power of the moon, we see clearly what to manifest and where to focus our attention. Each actionable step in the next lunar phase takes us closer to our dreams, achieving the life we so desire.

CHAPTER 10

WAXING MOON

The waxing moon is a beautiful and glistening reminder that the only constant in life is change (thank you to Greek philosopher Heraclitus). As the moon starts to smile with that silver curve, we are drawn into the waxing essences of enhancement, inspiration, commitment and new growth. As she grows after the new moon, you can feel yourself growing too, creating and attracting riches until the fullness lights up the sky.

The waxing moon has a magnetic energy to her, where you may find you, too, attract new opportunities into your everyday life. It's also a time for boldness and willpower, inviting you to focus on your new moon goals with determination, and a time to drive them forward. Now is the phase to put daily effort into the intentions set out during the new moon, whether that's through ritual or action. Success flows where your focus goes.

Setting a goal and taking action to achieve that goal can feel exciting and challenging. Our brains can see change as a threat, but when we work toward something, we have to change. We have to do things differently, or go through a rite of passage, so that our brains have the opportunity to grow.

It takes strength to step past any fearful thoughts and face any obstacles that arise from doing new things, but from that strength, resilience is born. And when we're resilient we can move through life with a deeper trust in our ability to cope.

When we take that action, get a bit uncomfortable, overcome the obstacles that crop up and grow in resilience, we can find joy in the uphill hike. Truly magical things unfold in us when we devote ourselves to something that is deeply aligned. You don't need pristine conditions to take the first step – nothing will ever be perfect or 100 per cent ready. And remember flexibility when you do move forward with your goals, as this will help you feel at peace with the natural ups and downs of life. Sometimes, however, quitting something is the only option, and there is much power in giving up something that no longer fits in with your inner world and values. Having said that, we're often capable of much more than we think.

A FEELING OF CALM

When bringing our goals to fruition, it's effective if we're centred and calm. To do this, we can activate our parasympathetic nervous system, responsible for calmness. The vagus nerve, which runs from the brainstem to the colon, counteracts stress and generates a relaxation response.

One way to stimulate the vagus nerve is to experience awe. This is an emotion that we feel in response to something vast, leading us to feel inspired and connected. This can be looking at a blood moon, being part of a heartening group or standing at the top of a mountain. Or it can happen much closer to home. Looking at the smallest details of nature creates a micro-awe that fills us with absolute wonderment – it's like a little mini mind earthquake. As we know, spending time in nature is beneficial to our wellbeing, but so is picturing yourself in a relaxing spot. Even if you can't get outside, imagining that you're on a blissful beach or in a moonlit forest will help put your body in a calmer state. Other ways to generate a relaxation response include meditation, yoga and listening to music.

THE CALMING POWER OF SPELLS

Spells, rituals, affirmations, prayer, yoga and meditation are all ways to help us feel connected. Connected to what? To your feelings, your desires, your body, your surroundings, the universe and, also to right here, you beauties – reading this book and performing the same spells, which will connect you all to one another, too.

Spells can be simple. Humming your favourite tune is a spell. Drinking tea in the morning and saying to yourself, "I feel grateful" is a spell. Savouring a walk in nature is a spell (especially if you chat to the trees – or is that just me?). Spells help you feel connected to the world around you, and also calm the amygdala in your brain, which is responsible for the flight or fight response. When we feel calm, we can experience greater clarity, which helps us with our intention-setting.

 ## Lunar ritual for prosperity and luck

Let's celebrate that feeling of awe by creating a rune stone. It's thought that runic inscriptions on rune stones hold magical powers dating back to medieval times. The Fehu symbol that we will draw here means new beginnings, energy, spiritual wealth, potential and fulfilment – all perfect for setting intentions. During the waxing moon, Fehu invites prosperity and luck.

Please collect ethically and responsibly, and never remove pebbles from a beach.

1. Go for walk in a beautiful natural space. Explore the tiny details of our world, such as the complex grid of veins on a leaf or the scaly bark of a tree. Immerse yourself in the mystery and harmony of the everyday world.
2. At some point in your walk, select a pebble or stone you're drawn to. Perhaps it's the colour or the texture, or something you can't describe. Study it in detail and give thanks to the ground and your stone for sharing the magic.
3. With a focused mind, return home with your stone in hand and draw the Fehu symbol onto your stone.

4. Hold your rune stone in your hand and meditate on your intentions for a few minutes.
5. Return to your day feeling connected and centred. You can use the same rune stone during every waxing moon phase to charge the energy (and limit your pebble collecting.)

As the moon grows toward fullness, we move toward actionable change. Opportunities infused with .magic may flow, and we can't help but use them to our advantage. A sprinkle of courage and determination will help you make the most of your opportunities and bring about the shifts you would like to see.

CHAPTER 11

FULL MOON

About 15 days after the new moon, we see the full moon illuminate the sky. Casting a spell over the landscape, she is captivating. It's little wonder that moon goddesses have been revered since long ago. From Rhiannon, who was born during the first rise of the moon, to Selene, the goddess of the moon in Greek mythology, who would visit dreamers with answers to their questions, there are many lunar deities woven throughout our mythical history.

How do you feel when you look at the full moon? If you find solace in the moon, you might be a selenophile – someone who is fascinated by the moon. It's a word I love to shoehorn into most conversations! I see the moon as a symbol of our all-knowing energies. Always there, actively listening but never judging. Divinely appreciating your most hidden parts so you might do the same. With her inescapable brightness, the full moon tends to haul everything to the surface. Like a mirror, we have nowhere to hide underneath her gaze.

If you feel in flow with your life and intentions, you may feel a sense of fullness or completeness with the moon's peak energy. If so, you might enjoy a lovely satisfaction or sense of achievement during this phase, especially if you've been working toward your goals.

On the flip side, if you've been bottling things up, the full moon has a way of raising the curtain on those underlying worries and fears. She's asking us to face up to those unhealed parts of ourselves, moving away from the ego and toward a place of self-compassion.

TAKE ADVANTAGE OF THE FULL MOON

The full moon is a catalyst for healing. This isn't a time to overextend yourself though, as the intensity may lead to depletion or a moon "hangover" – a "moonover" as I like to call it. Self-care is vital at this time, especially if you're a highly sensitive person.

The full moon is the moment for deepest reflection, so it's a good idea to focus on what is working for you and what isn't. And perhaps avoid new projects during this time; it might go all kinds of wrong if you embark on something meaty without a clear head.

 Full moon writing prompts

As you wonder about your lunar journey at the time of the full moon, take time to ask yourself these questions.

- What is there to celebrate about your month so far?
- Is there anything you would do differently?
- What's calling for completion?
- What would you like to let go of?
- Did you showcase your talents?

- Did someone else's power overshadow you?
- Did you act according to or against your intuition, and how did this work out for you?
- Which of your new moon intentions are coming true?

With this full moon reflection, we are being asked to tend to ourselves with extra care and devotion. We can only shed our old skin and feel deserving of our desires if we show ourselves unconditional kindness.

Lunar spell: transformation

Around the time of the full moon, we can shine a spotlight on our wounds and transform old fears through the healing power of water. Water symbolizes flow and receptivity, which means it can help clear negative blocks and absorb intentions. We can work with water in our spells by creating some moon water. Moon water is simply water that has been energetically "charged" by the moon. Because the moon is at its most potent when it's full, this is the perfect time to craft a spell.

You will need:
- water, tap or filtered
- glass, jar or container
- rose quartz crystals
- cinnamon sticks
- mugwort leaves, dried

1. First, make some moon water. Pour 1 cup of water into a clean container. Add rose quartz crystals or some herbs, such as cinnamon or mugwort, if you have some. Stir gently.

2. Put the jar in the garden or on a windowsill for a few hours or overnight to charge the water with the moon's energy.
3. Carve out some time to perform your spell in the right space for you. Open your jar and say your full name out loud.
4. With your left hand, dip a finger or two into your moon water and anoint between your eyebrows at your third eye. As you do, say out loud,

"I see my dreams coming to life and my limitations setting free."

5. Next, anoint the base of your throat and say, "I let go of stagnant energy and call for transformations".

"I let go of stagnant energy and call for transformations."

6. Lastly, anoint your chest and say out loud, "My heart's desires are worthwhile and I work to release my fears".

"My heart's desires are worthwhile and I work to release my fears."

7. After the spell, you can add the moon water to your bath for a full moon bath ritual or put it on your altar for the rest of your day to honour this powerful lunar phase.

If the full moon had a love language, it would be acts of service. She shows up fully to guide us into a place of awareness. We're afforded this sacred moment each month to celebrate what we have and identify what doesn't fulfil us. She is our cosmic guiding light that shows the way even in dark times.

The full moon insights guide us on our spiritual path as we retreat into surrender during the next lunar phase.

CHAPTER 12

WANING MOON

After the full moon, the pearl in the sky starts to diminish until we eventually return to the darkness of the new moon. Our patterns have been brought to light under the full moon, and now the waning moon welcomes release and retreat.

It's a time to learn from your mistakes and collect insight about the way you work. As the shadow creeps further across the moon's surface, we have the chance to face inward and sit in the gap for a while. Without the need to push ahead, you can take a quiet moment to assess what's getting in your way. This is the time to release what was never yours to feel.

FEELINGS OF IMPOSTER SYNDROME

Often, that feeling of "imposter syndrome" can reach a peak during the waning moon. Feelings of inadequacy can lead us to, either avoid our new moon intentions, or undermine the value of our achievements, if we have made progress. We may feel incompetent or fraudulent in some way. This can lead us to falsely believe that everyone else is somehow better or "more than", bringing about physical and emotional symptoms.

Imposter syndrome can be a result of growing up in an environment where a child's outcome was overly praised, or when there were high levels of conflict with little support. The waning moon is a chance for us to do some work on ourselves and resolve some of our limiting behaviours. By reframing thoughts and building each other up as a female collective, we can dispel those old self-sabotage thoughts and choose a different path.

Imposter syndrome can happen within any age, gender, class or racial demographic, but research shows that people from marginalized groups are more likely to feel like an outsider due to prejudice and discrimination. If this is the case, imposter syndrome is caused by others and not by inherent beliefs.

No one is the fully realized version of "perfection". How would we ever grow and learn if this was the case? When you feel the sensations of imposter syndrome, and it's OK that you do, it actually means that you're pushing yourself beyond your usual limits. And that's a good thing. Incredible, in fact.

Instead of beating yourself up for having any feelings of self-doubt, remind yourself that you're amazing for even being here in the first place. You're increasing your abilities every time you experience imposter syndrome because you've pushed yourself out of your comfort zone, and that's something to feel great about. If things don't always go to plan, lean into gratitude for that learning experience. You always have something to give, even if it's not perfect or "better than". In our practice, we look at how we can move forward from imposter syndrome.

Lunar ritual: releasing and moving on

The waning moon calls us to release old patterns to make space for new ways of thinking and being. Sometimes, we need to mentally take ourselves out of negativity to visualize

MOON SEASONS

Something we can be sure of, is that our one faithful moon, which is beautiful at 4.46 billion years old, looks a little different every night. As you may know, the moon orbits the earth and the earth orbits the sun, and lunar phases are caused by the relative positions of the sun, moon and earth. The moon takes 27.3 days to complete one orbit around the earth and 29.5 days to change from new moon to new moon again, completing nearly 13 lunar cycles each year. Not only does she influence our oceans, but she also stabilizes our seasons of the year.

Because the moon rotates, we only ever see one side of the moon, but depending on where we call home, we will see the phases differently. The four main phases are:

- new moon
- waxing moon
- full moon
- waning moon

In the northern hemisphere, we see the moon get bigger (wax) from the right until it reaches the full moon and get smaller (wane) to the left, until the new moon. In the southern hemisphere, we see the moon wax from the left until it reaches the full moon, and get smaller (wane) to the right, until the new moon.

The new moon occurs when it is located between the earth and the sun and for this reason, can't be seen in the sky at this time. The full moon happens when it's on the opposite side of the sun with the earth in the middle. Because our moon doesn't shine, but simply reflects sunlight, its sphere is completely visible from the earth at that point.

how things can be different. This self-commitment ritual helps us live the idea of change for a few moments. A future pacing exercise, like this, allows us see the wonderful benefits of feeling valuable and lovable. This helps us move on from feelings of imposter syndrome and low self-confidence. To open up to intentional change, we can prepare ourselves with some moon breathing, which calms the nervous system.

1. First, let's try moon breathing, to help you feel calm and centred. To do this, close off your right nostril with your right thumb and breathe in through your left nostril. Notice the pause at the end of the inhale.
2. Now, close your left nostril with the fourth finger of your right hand, letting go of the thumb from your right nostril. Breathe out through the right nostril. Repeat a few times, breathing in through the left and out through the right, each time. Close your eyes, as you settle into this. When you feel more relaxed, allow your breath to return to a regular pattern and rest your hands in your lap.
3. Now bring your imagination to the fore. Imagine yourself at a crossroads somewhere. There is a fork to the left and a fork to the right. You can see a full-length mirror at the end of each path. You're about to explore both paths.
4. First, you take the left-hand path. When you get to the end, you see a future image of yourself in the mirror. This image is you in two years' time, if you continue to hold onto any feelings of self-doubt. Look at that for a while. Perhaps you're tired, unhappy, regretful?
5. Come back to the crossroads when you're ready. Next, you take the right-hand path. When you get to the end, you see a future image of yourself in two years' time. In the mirror,

see yourself looking vibrant and full of energy. You've worked on feeling valued and deserving.

6. As you watch your future self, radiating with positivity, the figure turns to you and says: "You can release your past regrets. You are deserving of a positive future".

7. You push the mirror glass, and like a door, it opens onto a beautifully inviting path. Imagine that you're excited about taking those first steps and are committed to a journey of self-empowerment. There will be twists and turns along the path, and you are ready to embrace them.

8. When you are ready, flutter your eyes open, taking this positive mindset forward as you return to your day.

The healing touch of the waning moon brings closure and change. As the moon finally fades from view, we flow back into the new moon, ready to transform old wounds into positive intentions. And so, the cycle begins again. Next, we travel into our most personal and possibly most powerful cyclical teacher: the menstrual cycle.

PART FOUR

MENSTRUAL CYCLE

Spiralling into our most intimate cycle, we create a heart-to-heart with our bodies in this next part of the book. You will go on a menstrual exploration, flowing through the four inner menstrual seasons, with the help of physical, emotional and spiritual guidance sessions to support and restore the mind, body and soul.

Each menstrual phase of your cycle brings about a set of strengths and a nest of opportunities to empower your healing journey and uncover the deepest levels of inner power.

These self-care sessions help you connect with, and place trust in, your cycle in a way that blends with the realistic demands of the outside world.

Life can be tough. Cost of living, burnout, social media politics, systemic injustices and uncertainty about the future are all very real. These nourishing sessions equip you with the practices and awareness needed to curate and live your life according to your natural cyclicality, liberating you to feel safe and whole.

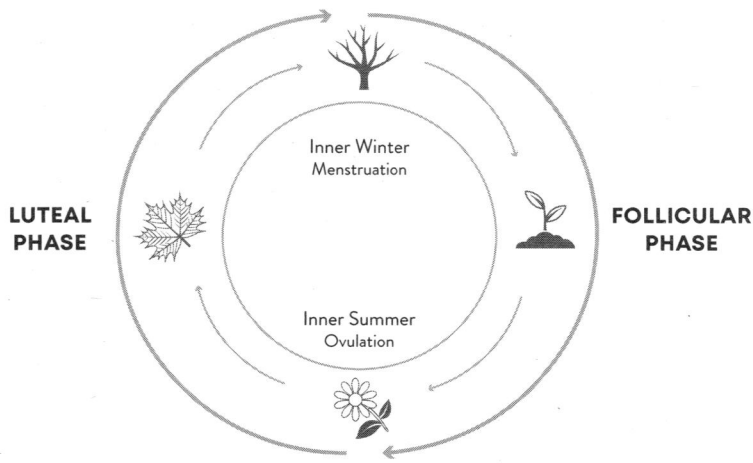

In the four menstrual chapters – inner spring, summer, autumn and winter – we begin with physical support, circle into emotional self-care and finish with rituals and practices to nourish our spiritual selves.

There's also no pressure to get it "right" or do any of this perfectly. We're moving away from the urgency for women to appear like they're coping and can do it all (thank you, patriarchy), and instead, be at ease with exploring our own strengths, vulnerabilities and needs more deeply.

To get the most out of these healing practices and tips, it may be worth charting your menstrual cycle. There are many ways to do this, whether you like to use an app on your phone or prefer journaling your thoughts, feelings and energy levels each day of your cycle – or both.

Let's take day 1 as the first day of your bleed. You can start charting on that day, or begin now if you've got a feeling about where in your cycle you may be. This will give you a starting point to help you to notice the moon phase, the external season and where you are in your life cycle to optimize the cyclical adventure. Please note this book will begin with our spring season, which starts on approximately day six of your cycle.

This menstrual voyage is for anyone who bleeds, regardless of gender. If you are postmenopausal, you can use these insights to understand those in your life who have a cycle. It's also an opportunity to reflect on your menstrual journey, deepening your feminine power and healing any wounds. The gifts of growth and renewal now sit in the seasons of the earth and the phases of the moon.

Tracking your menstrual cycle has so many benefits:

- You get a heads-up when you're about to enter the luteal phase (hello PMS)
- You will also get to know the length of your cycle (many of us do not have a 28-day cycle)
- You will start to notice how you experience the four menstrual phases.

In the book *Wild Power*, Red School authors and pioneers, Alexandra Pope and Sjanie Hugo Wurlitzer (see Further Reading) refer to the process of menstrual cycle embodiment as:

"The culmination of wisdom that you begin to live by, the peace that you make with who you are, and the freedom to express your creativity in the world".

Your menstrual phases are a gorgeous portal to deeper self-healing and a way to develop trust in your body again.

HORMONAL CONTRACEPTION AND HRT

I'm not someone who disapproves of anyone taking birth control, whether that's to prevent pregnancy or help control hormonal imbalances. We all do what we need to do. I had the contraception injection for many years before having children. For people with severe menstrual symptoms, it can feel like the only way to resolve some of the suffering.

That said, it is worth taking time to understand the potential effects of birth control. Synthetic hormones prevent the natural surges of oestrogen and progesterone, making awareness of your menstrual cycle tricky. In our context of working with our flow, this can mean reduced opportunities for emotional and spiritual personal growth. Hormonal birth control can deplete certain nutrients in the gut (especially B vitamins) and can increase the stress response.

If you take the pill and still menstruate, it will be a "breakthrough bleed" rather than a natural period. As no ovulation will usually occur while taking contraception (but it can happen, so be aware), the bleeding is simply a withdrawal from the hormones in the contraception. That being said, you can still work with the cycle you do have, noting down how you feel according to which day you are on.

There are non-hormonal contraception options such as the diaphragm, copper IUD and condoms if you're looking to explore other options. Please be aware that condoms are the only option to prevent sexually transmitted diseases (STDs).

If you're happy to stay on hormonal birth control, feel like it's the only option for now or have a menstrual condition (see below) that results in irregular or absent periods, you can still work with lunar period tracking. You can mark day one when it's the new moon and work with the main energies of each lunar phase as the month unfolds.

If you are peri-menopausal and taking sequential combined Hormone Replacement Therapy (HRT), it's common to experience a withdrawal bleed at the end of your cycle.

Let's look at how the four moon phases align with the four menstrual phases to give you a cyclical anchor.

- **New Moon** = Menstruation/Winter = Connection, rest, inner guidance, self-care.
- **Waxing Moon** = Follicular/Spring = Motivation, rising energy, focus, assertiveness.

- **Full Moon** = Ovulation/Summer = Visibility, self-love, celebration, desire, expression.
- **Waning Moon** = Luteal/Autumn = Inner critic, discernment, retreat, reflection.

MENSTRUAL CONDITIONS

Many menstrual conditions can affect your cycle. The emphasis in this book is how to live in flow with your seasons, but if you need more specific advice on how to improve your menstrual health on a body and nutritional level, I would recommend *You Can Have a Better Period* by Le'Nise Brothers. She talks about our menstrual cycle being considered the body's fifth vital sign, giving us information about what's normal and what isn't. If you'd like to know more about the emotional root causes of certain menstrual conditions, I would recommend the online workshop *The Wisdom of Your Cycle* by Tracey Stevens. Please see a doctor if you're concerned about your cycle. Here are some common conditions that can impact our cycles:

- **Endometriosis:** A painful condition affecting at least one in ten women of reproductive age. Cells similar to those in the uterus lining are also found in other areas of the body, including the pelvis, bowels and legs.
- **Adenomyosis:** Tissue that grows in the lining of the womb grows into the muscle in the wall of the uterus.
- **Fibroids:** Affecting many women (and disproportionately black women), these are benign tumours made up of smooth muscle cells and fibrous tissue that develop in or around the womb.

- **Ovarian cysts:** Fluid-filled sacs that develop on an ovary. They usually go away naturally and don't cause symptoms unless they are too big or rupture, in which case they can disrupt the cycle.
- **Polycystic ovary syndrome (PCOS):** A common condition affecting roughly one in ten women. The ovaries produce too many androgens (male hormones), preventing ovulation from taking place.
- **Amenorrhea:** A missed period for several consecutive months, which isn't a result of pregnancy or breastfeeding but hormonal imbalances or health-related issues, such as stress or disordered eating.
- **Menorrhagia:** Heavy menstrual bleeding (changing your sanitary towel or tampon hourly) or prolonged bleeding (that lasts more than seven days) as a result of fibroids, hormone imbalances, PCOS or pelvic inflammatory disease.
- **Dysmenorrhea:** Moderate to severe pain during the menstrual cycle, which is usually located in the lower abdomen but can spread to the lower back and thighs.
- **Premenstrual syndrome (PMS):** Symptoms experienced during the luteal phase of their menstrual cycle, including mood swings, anxiety, fatigue, breast tenderness and changes to skin, hair, appetite and sex drive.
- **Premenstrual dysphoric disorder (PMDD):** More intense PMS symptoms that carry greater negative repercussions, such as joint or muscle pain, depression and, in some cases, suicidal thoughts.

We have the power to improve our menstrual experiences. Tuning into the needs of our mind, body and soul gives us a place to belong, making us feel happier and fulfilled.

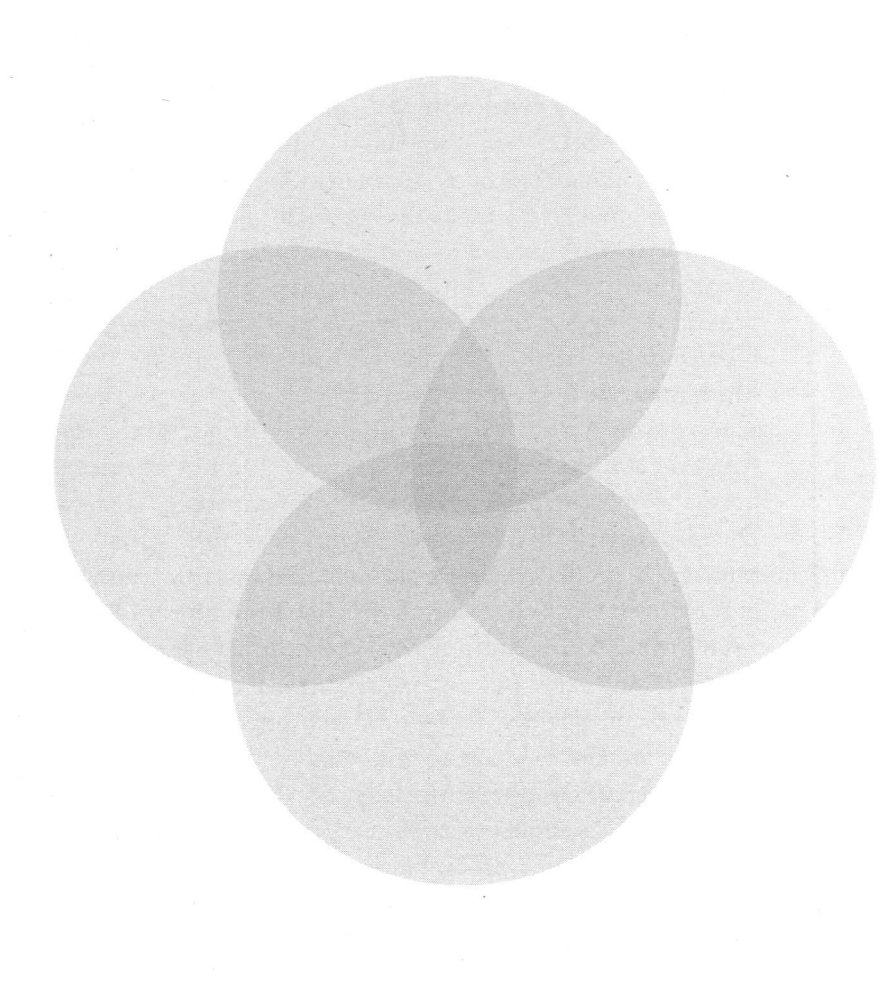

CHAPTER 13

INNER SPRING

Come in, friends.

Let's flow into our menstrual seasons, starting with inner spring. Inner spring, or pre-ovulation, makes an appearance soon after menstruation has finished, usually between days 6–11 (if you have a 28-day cycle).

Growth and potential are our spring beacons. Now, the uterine lining starts to replenish, with increasing oestrogen so that a potential fertilized egg can implant. Emotionally, there's a playful, rising energy that allows us to sprout new ideas and feel motivated after the cocoon of menstruation has ended. Spiritually, we're thickening our ability to align our growing strengths with a sense of purpose. This is a phase of many changes on many levels.

Inner spring mimics the emerging energies of the waxing moon, where we feel energized to achieve goals and feel assertive in doing so.

The inner spring superpowers are: curiosity, adventure, productivity, optimism, focus, renewal and strength. How might this look in the everyday world? It can mean sharper focus, motivation to take on new projects and spontaneity to try different experiences.

Your renewed enthusiasm for life can pave the way for you to be seen and heard, making it the ideal moment to take up extra space in the outside world. You may feel physically and emotionally stronger after your period has ended, allowing you to take more on and feel resilient in the process.

As you open up after menstruation, you're able to cherish the little things, feeling hopeful about your life and what you have to offer. This makes it a lovely time to relish new starts and set intentions for the month ahead.

As with each of the four menstruation phases, there's a trickier side. Sometimes, the urge to be finished with the "inconvenience" of menstruation, and fit in with outer-world standards, can feel so pressing that we don't allow ourselves to unfurl gently into the spring phase. I hear you.

Affording yourself a breath of tenderness will help you unfold your spring energy at a rhythm that suits you. Your spring days are sweet and precious. They invite you to toy with possibility and take time to dream big. Feel free to be experimental and playful, trying out new things and taking risks when you feel inclined to.

Saying a (sometimes unavoidable) "yes" to the world without a protective layer can make us feel at odds. We might end up rejecting our vulnerable side, even though that's the slice others appreciate most.

Busyness has become our world's gold medal; if we can prove our efforts are in great demand, we must matter. And with a wing and a prayer, we might just be able to get it all done, but we're risking too much here. We can end up being disorganized, overly competitive and a bit self-centred if we get too serious in spring.

Something (or someone) could throw us off or cut us down if our inner spring is too driven. As the seasonal, lunar and life cycles steadily build resilience, your inner seasons require the same. If you resonate with this, it isn't a beat-yourself-up opportunity, but a foxy way to resolve obstacles and feel more in tune with your needs.

VULNERABILITY

Vulnerability is one of our biggest strengths. It allows us to take risks and create opportunities. The courage it takes to be vulnerable allows us to accept our imperfections. Being seen for who we really are gives us a deep sense of worthiness. This builds self-confidence and helps us face challenges despite their uncertainty. Uncertainty is really the only thing we can be certain about in life! In this vulnerable place, new skills and strengths are born. Creativity, flexibility, resilience and compassion empower us to reach our true potential and connect with others more deeply.

The self-care sessions that follow are conscious acts to help you embody health on a physical, emotional and spiritual level. When we get our physical bodies on board, we can care for our emotional and spiritual selves more easily.

PHYSICAL HEALING

Starting with the basics, inner spring is the proliferative phase, which occurs from the end of your period until ovulation. Proliferative simply means growing; the uterus lining grows so an egg can implant into it. The bit between your bleed and ovulation is known as the follicular phase. During the follicular phase, the pituitary gland in the brain releases FSH (follicle-stimulating hormone), which tells the ovaries to produce several follicles.

As the ovarian follicles get bigger, they produce oestrogen (or estradiol), which builds the womb lining in preparation for fertilization. One of these follicles continues to grow while the others degenerate, looking after the maturing egg within it. This egg will then be released during ovulation.

Whether we're looking to conceive or simply optimize our wellbeing, we need our lovely spring phase to be as healthy as possible. When we look after our needs by eating good food, sleeping well and listening to the body's wishes, we support the rising hormones and encourage a healthy ovulation. How can we optimize this phase at a body level?

 ## Sleep on it

This is the time in your cycle that you're most likely to get a good dose of sleep. The duration of REM (rapid eye movement) sleep is higher in the follicular phase, which helps us with memory and mood. Oestrogen is also responsible for body temperature regulation; you're more able to feel cool and comfortable at night.

During this phase, you might feel and be more active, and this increased physicality can also make it easier for you to rest at night. However, avoid late-night gym sessions as higher intensity movement can make it harder for the brain to wind down.

 ## Nourish yourself

Approaching your nutrition with a cyclical approach is a beautiful way to develop a sense of trust and natural flow in the way you eat. Oestrogen starts to rise during our inner spring, so our energy levels will naturally increase. What we don't want to happen is there to be an excess of oestrogen, causing an imbalance in our hormones. Fermented foods (think kefir or kombucha) and cruciferous veggies can be a lovely way to keep your oestrogen levels in check.

Eating good fats, such as avocados and olives, and increasing protein-rich foods, such as chicken, beans, pulses and eggs, is nourishing here. Eggs are also a great source of vitamin B12, which is needed for healthy ovulation.

At this time of the month, you may be drawn to lighter foods like salads and smoothies. This is linked to the fact that oestrogen is a natural appetite suppressant. However, remember your protein – sprinkling some seeds and nuts onto your salads is an easy way to ensure you aren't forgetting the crucial nutrients needed for a healthy spring.

OESTROGEN AND FASTING

Fasting can help balance oestrogen dominance (look out for mood swings) or oestrogen deficiency (think peri symptoms).

There are many other reported benefits to fasting, such as reduced inflammation, decreased risk of diseases, cellular repair and better cognitive performance. However, most of the research has been carried out on either men or mice, so unfortunately we're lacking in evidence of what fasting might mean for women. We could write a whole book on gender bias in scientific research, but for now, we'll stick to the essentials.

If you're going to do a fast, and I do on occasion, it may be best if you do it in this spring phase. As you may not feel as hungry in this phase, fasting can feel easier.

Please note that fasting should be avoided during the progesterone-dominant phases (days 20–28) of the menstrual cycle. If you have a history of disordered eating, are pregnant or breastfeeding, have diabetes, are taking certain medications or are deemed too young, fasting is not advised.

 ## Skin love

Rising oestrogen levels can mean a growing glow with an increase in collagen production. This may make your skin look plump, dewy and elastic a few days into this phase. Your skin may feel less greasy too. As your skin may be less sensitive, this can be a good time to try that new skincare product if desired. It can also be a good time to gently exfoliate your skin as new skin cells form with the increase in collagen and hyaluronic acid, so you'll be double-charging the turnover process. As always, work out what products work best for your skin, especially when it comes to exfoliation.

Nourishing food and a good skincare routine will also help to care for your skin. However, it's important not to get too emotionally hung up on the outcomes. Skin "neutrality" is about moving away from either feeling positive or negative about your skin. Adopting a neutral take on your skin is a way to both embody self-acceptance and reject the patriarchal culture of needing to "look good" all the time. Yes!

 ## Vulva low-down

What can you expect to experience in your vulva and vagina during inner spring? In general, you know what's normal for you. Noticing how your body changes throughout the month can help you know what to expect. You might find that your cervix produces more mucus alongside the rising oestrogen levels, which can be a milky white colour and either thick or creamy in consistency.

Or you may feel a bit dry in the early part of the spring phase. Vaginal dryness, in general, is more common during the perimenopausal years but can happen to anyone with a vulva, at any age. A natural, organic lubricant may help during sex. You may find that you produce more natural lubrication toward the end of spring when you approach ovulation.

 ## Sex and intimacy

Arousal and oestrogen are best pals, with oestrogen increasing sexual desire and lubricating vaginal tissues. With each passing spring day, you may find your passion rises with an itch to connect with your other(s) in a sensual way.

Many women find that their desire for sex increases during the spring phase, as oestrogen and testosterone levels are high. If you're not a fan of period sex, you might feel ready soon after your bleed ends.

Touch releases oxytocin (the love hormone) for women, which helps us to feel trusting and develop romantic attachments, so you may want to get closer to your partner during this phase.

 ## Exercise

As with everything else, your cycle can affect the way you exercise. With the rising oestrogen during the follicular phase, you can up the intensity of your workouts a little, if you choose to. Increasing levels of oestrogen can help us build muscle mass, so lifting weights and strength training can work well, during this phase.

Incorporating cardio work into your exercise routine capitalizes on spring upgrades in energy output and motivation. As you're a bit more experimental during this time, feel free to try out a new class to keep things fresh.

Using your menstrual cycle to get the most out of your exercise routine is a growing area of research. Any movement that feels good to you right now, is good. Essentially, you are the expert of your own body so always tailor things to your needs.

PLAYFUL YOGA POSE

Flip your world upside down with a playful yoga inversion to help you see things from a new perspective, and stretch your whole body in the process.

You will need:
- yoga mat or non-slip floor
- loose, comfortable clothing

1. Stand straight with your legs as wide as it's comfortable for them to be.
2. Exhale, as you fold over, with a flat back, reaching down the outside of your legs or onto the floor (wherever feels comfortable to you). There's no need to push yourself and there are no prizes here, so just go down as far as feels right without rounding your back.

3. If it feels good, fold a little deeper on each exhale.
4. Let your head hang loose. Take this moment to wonder about the joy of the upside-down world for a few moments.
5. When ready to move out of the position, spread your arms or place them on your hips and slowly rise on the inhale. Come back feeling refreshed and relaxed.

EMOTIONAL HEALING

We may feel playful, curious, determined and spontaneous throughout our inner spring phase. Or we may find stepping out into the world outside intimidating, rushed and a bit alienating. A bit of both, perhaps.

Dipping into the world of cyclical emotions can help us understand ourselves with greater clarity so that we can live with a greater sense of balance and ease. So, let's get curious!

 Curiosity writing prompts

When we get curious, we can resolve inner conflict more easily and really see life's potential ahead of us. Take a moment now to ask yourself the following questions:

- What recent achievements do you feel good about?
- How would you like to spend some of your free time?
- What fascinates you and how can you learn more about it?
- What effort are you putting into your needs and desires?

- How do you feel about new beginnings?
- How do you protect your energy?
- What is your version of success?
- When do you feel playful? What stops you from letting go?
- How do you feel about vulnerability?
- When do you feel stubborn and why?
- What would you try if there were no negative outcomes?

Relationships spring clean

This is the loveliest phase to spring-clean our relationships. Your inner spring strengths of curiosity and spontaneity can restore fresh, playful vibes to your most meaningful relationships, whether these are romantic or otherwise.

Firstly, make a plan to do something fun with your friends, family and/or partner. This can be in the next few days or perhaps arrange something for the inner spring season next month. When you're oh-so entertaining and have more energy to invest in people, connections will feel re-energized and soul-lifting.

Catching up, laughing out loud and maintaining plenty of eye-contact help cultivate a feeling of appreciation for each other. If it's a romantic relationship you're working on, surprising them with something new creates mystery and suspense. This is vital to relationship longevity.

Secondly, look at the parts of your relationship/s that can hold it back from being nourishing. Instead of stockpiling negativity or complaints, which can lead to feelings of contempt, try saying what you need to say with honesty and integrity.

As your curiosity will be enhanced during inner spring, you will be less likely to feel defensive when talking things through. This can help you work together and even feel excited about solving any relationship hurdles.

 ## Self-love: forgiveness

Spring loves a quick win, but we can learn to stop polishing ourselves to "perfection". Our wonderful spring qualities of determination and drive are admirable, yet we don't need to be the "final version" to be valuable and lovable. The art of self-forgiveness and compassion, when things don't go to plan, gives way to a fulfilling spring.

Spring calls for us to build a sense of stability and resilience but with vulnerability and curiosity as the cornerstones of self-love.

As we're more likely to give things a go in this menstrual phase, we must afford ourselves the chance to mess it up a little, and this looks a lot like forgiving ourselves for our mistakes. Loving yourself in the way that you need is a deserving and worthwhile pursuit. And what better way to do this than to write yourself notes or a letter of kindness? If this feels a bit weird or silly, it might be one you really can't skip. Trust me, it's a healing and cathartic experience.

You will need:
- sticky notes, paper or journal
- pen/s

1. Write a few (or many) words of compassion, reflecting on any negative and unloving self-beliefs. For example:

Negative self-belief	Positive self-belief
Not getting it right	I do the best I can
Not getting it perfect	I learn and grow each day
Not being enough	I add value to the world
Being too much or too little	I accept myself fully
Not matching up to others	I appreciate my unique gifts

This will help you reframe any spring judgement and invite self-love into your being.

2. Now try writing a letter to yourself. This may flow more easily if you can imagine it's said from the perspective of a nurturing friend and written in the third person e.g. "I'm sorry for telling you you're not enough by keeping you so very busy. You are full of potential and are capable of achieving your every dream."

3. Now add to the letter, filling the page with love and tenderness. Say how you are so worthy, appreciated and valued, expressing complete and unconditional love and respect. For example:

- I'm proud of you because …
- I admire you for …
- I am grateful for …
- I think you're amazing because …

4. Once you have written your letter, re-read it until the words really sink in. You can either keep the letter or safely burn it to symbolize moving forward with renewed positivity.

BOX BREATHING

In spring, we can feel like we have to get everything done. Making time for some gentle breaths can help us let go of that pressure to rush things through, helping you feel refreshed and recharged. It's a lovely way to start the day or to take a pause in your working, active day.

1. Find a safe space to relax, either sitting, standing or lying down, and close your eyes, or keep your eyes open, with a soft gaze in front of you.
2. Inhale for a count of four, allowing your abdomen to rise as you breathe in.
3. Pause at the end of the inhale for four beats.
4. Exhale gently for four, releasing the air steadily from your lungs. Allow your abdomen to fall gently as you do so.
5. Pause at the end of the exhale for four beats. Repeat for as long as you need to feel calmer and more grounded.

Cold water swimming

In your spring season, you have a lowered sensitivity to the cold, so this is a great time to try cold water swimming. The benefits of cold, outdoor swimming include reduced inflammation, improved cognition and increased gratitude.

Being outside in a blue space encourages mindfulness and good mental health. Cold water is also amazing for perimenopausal symptoms, such as anxiety and hot flushes. Here are a few tips to encourage you to dip your toes in the water:

1. Find a space geared up for cold water swimming, such as a lido or lake, and speak to the organizer/s before attending, as some might require advance booking or safety training first.
2. Choose a good weather day, ideally with sunshine! Don't start cold water swimming when it's really cold outside.
3. Make sure you have the right kit, like a wetsuit. Some venues hire these out.
4. Go with a friend for moral support and safety – as well as fun!
5. Listen to your body and only dip or swim for a short time while you get used to it.
6. Make sure you keep moving to keep warm.
7. Breathe deeply with some slow, long breaths when you first enter the water and give yourself a moment or two to feel the cold before slowly getting all the way in.
8. After your dip, keep yourself warm and dry with cozy clothes and a hat.

Make sure it's safe for you to take part in this practice. Heart conditions, pregnancy, high blood pressure and breathing difficulties mean it might not be for you – please check with your doctor first.

OUT-OF-THE-BOX MEDITATION

Meditation has many benefits, including helping you feel peaceful and developing self-compassion. If you meditate every day, even if it's just for a short while, your brain learns to pace itself (through neuroplasticity), and you can extend that ability to regulate your emotions and feel more centred in everyday life. Instead of getting in a spin, we learn to be calm, allowing creativity and joy to flow.

To fulfil the wholeness of spring, we can hear out the messages of our gut. When we overthink (and spring loves a bit of rationalization), we can shut ourselves off from important internal signals and out-of-the-box thinking.

Aligning rationality and intuition can bring our inner spring into balance and stop things from being too one-sided. So, let's try this simple meditation together:

- Close your eyes and place your hands on your stomach.
- Tune in and simply allow your breath to flow in and out. Whatever your gut has to say to you is valid, here. Simply listen for a few minutes.
- Understanding the messages of your intuition will allow a steady flow of vitality and power to grow. There is no set way of doing this. Sit with your inner space for as long as you need.
- When you're ready, bring awareness back into the room and open your eyes.

SPIRITUAL HEALING

Seeking out mystical practices from long ago connects us to a sense of oneness and gives us a feeling of belonging. Moving even further into our spring phase, we can develop a sacred and intimate relationship with our spiritual selves. Let me tell you a story:

FOLKTALE STORY: RHIANNON

Old stories are powerful. They are a way to ground us in the essence of who we are through the lens of imagining something bigger than ourselves. Who are we becoming in this passage of life and what unknown elements do we need to lose and gain along the way? Let's turn to Rhiannon for spiritual inspiration.

Rhiannon was a fairy queen who ruled the sun, pulling it across the sky every day. She was associated with horses, forgiveness, resilience, rest, communication and abundance. Rhiannon was also connected to the Otherworld: a mystical realm that exists beyond the boundaries of the material world.

Rhiannon was so very charming that everyone, including her husband, Pwyll, instantly fell in love with her. Rhiannon made Pwyll wait for her, and despite appearing to ride on her white horse slowly when they met, she was impossible to catch – unless, of course, she allowed it. She demonstrated both playfulness and strategic expertise during their time together.

Later, Rhiannon was wrongly accused of killing their son. She spent seven years imprisoned, where she would share her story to all that approached. Rhiannon was eventually set free, returning to the palace as a great queen.

This goddess reminds us of the inner spring energy of wanting to get things moving where they may have been held captive. And that sometimes, we are being paced by something mysterious and powerful, without knowing that it may lead to greater opportunities.

This story speaks of our resilience, even when we're vulnerable, and motivates us to share our stories to be truly seen. Through Rhiannon's tale, we learn that, with an appreciation for life, we can move forward stronger than ever by aligning our strengths with our divinity.

Self-expression: your story

We have explored a story from the past. Now, how about your story? Inner spring is all about purpose. Inviting ourselves to connect with the outer world with the two fundamental strengths of vulnerability and power is a pathway to wholehearted expression.

When we get to the bottom of it all, our purpose is simply to share our truest selves and have the space for this to be seen. This can look like many things, depending on who you are and what you want to show. Our next self-care session can help you connect with your purpose by sharing your unique story.

You will need:
- paper or a journal
- pen/s

1. Write at the top of your page the title: "My story is gorgeous and unlike any others because ..."
2. Without stopping and over-thinking, write freely for five minutes, inspired by this prompt. The healing is in the act of writing your personal story. It's a lovely idea to keep it somewhere safe in case you need reminding of your awesomeness in the future.

 Crystals: set your intentions

With feelings of inner seasonal renewal, we can look to crystals to support our spiritual experience. Crystals are thought to possess powerful healing powers when their vibrations interact with our individual energetic frequency. They are often part of ancient practices to empower, protect and heal people.

Meditating with a crystal can "supercharge" things, especially in connection to your purpose. When you set spring intentions with a crystal, you're collaborating with the universe to invite opportunities that line up with your commitments.

Emerald is a lovely crystal to work with during preovulation as it summons the natural vitality of this phase. Be sure to get your crystals from ethical sources and cleanse them by placing them in the sunlight for 20–30 minutes, if possible, before using them.

Try setting an inner spring intention with your emerald crystal by putting it in your hand and focusing on what you want, as though it's already happening. You can say something like: "I appreciate this (strength/abundance/relationship/etc.), harnessing the energy it brings for the greater good".

Womb ritual: yoni steam

Yoni steaming is an ancient practice used to cleanse wombs and reconnect with Mother Earth. It is believed to be an ancient indigenous healing practice not isolated to one origin.

It's thought to nourish reproductive health, relax vaginal tissues, relieve cramps, clear away stagnant brown blood and help with cysts, fibroids, prolapses or menstrual irregularities. Steaming has an "upwards" energy, supporting the spring-rising energy of intention-setting.

As you shouldn't steam during menstruation, it's a nourishing spring practice for renewal, following your period. The vagina is self-cleaning when it's in balance, so you don't have to do it, if this doesn't appeal, but steaming can be a great way to aid that natural process.

Always consult your doctor before steaming. Certain contraindications include pregnancy, postpartum, menstruation, IUD contraception, yeast infections or UTIs.

You will need:
- small saucepan or yoni bowl, that fits over a toilet
- fresh or dried yoni-safe herbs, such as raspberry leaves, basil, lavender, chamomile or rosemary (or buy a pre-made mix)

1. Pour about three cups of water into the pan, and bring to the boil.
2. Turn off the heat, stir in one cup or a small handful of yoni-safe herbs, and cover for three to five minutes. Allow the water to cool for another five minutes.

3. Steam for 15–20 minutes. You can do this by squatting over the pan in a comfortable position, with your forearms reaching in front of you on a cushion or bolster.
4. Meditate on what you would like to shed and what you would like to bring to life during your steam.
5. Afterwards, carefully pour the liquid and herbs away.

 ## Spring affirmations

Affirmations help you set guidelines to align your daily choices with your purpose. They calm the system and positively impact your vibrational energy, consolidating all the work you've been doing on yourself. You can say your affirmations whenever it feels right to connect with your true strengths:

I share my stories as a way to be truly seen.
I am both powerful and playful.
I connect with the outer world with curiosity and appreciation.
I can be both rational and intuitive.
I attract abundance and am generous with my fortunes.
I allow myself to take risks and forgive myself when they don't pay off.
I am comfortable with rising energy and embrace new beginnings.
I am successful and self-compassionate.

 ## Essential oil: lemongrass

Essential oils have been a part of spiritual practices throughout history, and a way to connect with, and heal, the body, mind and spirit. This life force energy is the very essence of the plant and carries a vibrational pattern. When we apply or burn essential oils, they, in turn, affect our frequency levels.

Lemongrass is our spring special someone. This essential oil can be used for spiritual healing as it aligns our inner self with our external world. It's also great for helping us to maintain self-control, stick to a plan, and dispel procrastination. Lemongrass is a holistic oil that brings clarity and purpose to our actions.

You can diffuse two to three drops of lemongrass essential oil in a diffuser to fill a room. Or add a few drops to water when washing floors to remove any bad luck present, and embrace a sense of newness in your space.

 Cosmic ceremony: purpose

Being seen and heard by a group of women, while in a sacred space of rest, is a way for us to feel connected and important. If you can, get together with your people and find a location that suits everyone. Weekly meetings can be something to look forward to and deepen a feeling of togetherness.

Purpose is the theme of this gathering. Purpose can show up in every season, as wanting our inner strengths to be seen by others is month-long, but now is a great time to focus on it. In your collective, chat about what it means to align your lives with a sense of purpose, and how it feels to be seen by other women. Feel free to chat beforehand to work out everyone's various needs and expectations. As a group, it's a good idea to ask yourself questions such as:

- What do you dream of?
- What does a meaningful life look like to you?
- What is the drive behind your aspirations?
- Where do you find inspiration?

INNER SPRING AND THE OTHER CYCLES

Get closer for a minute, lovelies.

Let's now look at how your inner seasons can be impacted by the three other ways of living cyclically: lunar, life and seasonal. We are all unique and it would be impossible to describe every possible variation of flow within each of you, but I can guide you on your path of self-discovery.

 ## Spring and the lunar cycle

How may your inner spring change, according to the phases of the moon? Let's take a look at each lunar phase, and what you might experience:

Spring and the new moon

Inner spring and the new moon can work well together, carving energetic space for possibility and manifestation. A new moon ritual can give your hopeful, "anything is possible" inner spring energies some extra shine. Seek to remember that divine pause during inner spring as this will help you integrate your self-development journey. Otherwise, you may lose sight of your path without a sacred breath.

Spring and the waxing moon

If you're in preovulation during the waxing moon phase, you may find that life feels sweet. You may experience new ideas and wonder at the beauty around you double-fold. However, it may also feel too driven if you're not keeping any shadow characteristics (see page 76) in check. Unfolding your spring energy gently will be your ally.

Spring and the full moon

With this cyclical blend, you may find that any unhealed parts of yourself come to a head. This can feel like many different things, but one can be a highlighted lack of fun or playfulness. The hamster wheel of getting to places fast can mean we forget our mischievousness, seeing seriousness too often. If so, factor in a little playtime, whatever that looks like for you.

Spring and the waning moon

When you're in spring and the moon is shrinking, you may have landed into a push-me-pull-me situation. The waning moon wants you to shed what no longer serves you and your inner spring wants you to set intentions of growth. This doesn't have to be an almighty inner brawl, but it is something to be aware of. You may need to face what no longer serves you before sowing new seeds.

MOON SPELL FOR RESILIENCE

As we're in the land of the moon, I have a lunar spell for you. Whatever moon phase you experience inner spring in, you will need resilience to help you move forward with energy.

You will need:
- a little jar or pot
- incense stick of your choosing
- lighter or matches
- paper
- pen
- salt
- dried lavender
- fresh or dried rose petals
- ground cinnamon
- blue candle

1. Cleanse your jar or pot by burning an incense stick and waving it inside like a wand for a few seconds.
2. Write down a note of resilience to yourself such as, "I bend but do not break" or "With the power of the Universe and the strength of my spirit, I grow strong".
3. Pour in salt to fill a quarter of your pot. Now add roughly the same quantity of dried lavender and rose petals.
4. Place your note on top, and sprinkle over a little cinnamon.
5. Put the lid on, then seal it shut by dripping wax from the blue candle onto it.
6. Place the jar on your altar or keep it on your bedside table. Allow the magic to do its work.

Spring and the yearly cycles

As with the lunar phases, your inner seasons can feel changeful depending on the yearly season you find yourself in. The seasons of the year can mirror how you feel, bring inner strengths to the fore or unveil parts of you that need extra love and attention. Exploring our inner and outer seasons helps us live more centred and joyful lives.

Inner spring and yearly spring

If you're in your inner spring and it's the external spring season, you may feel excited to move forward and make plans for sunnier times. If you feel impatience or frustration to get things moving, step more lightly. Life will blossom at the right time.

Inner spring and yearly summer

If it's warm outside and you're hoping to uncurl slowly from the wintery depths, make sure your inner spring doesn't get too hot too quickly ... or you may feel a bit parched with the extra heat. These two seasons may also enrich each other with their outwardly focused energy of showing up to the surrounding world.

Inner spring and yearly autumn

As autumn asks us to let go of things no longer needed, you can use this menstrual phase of deepened curiosity to wonder about what you've been holding onto. See the parts of you that you want to surrender, with the spring strengths of hopefulness and focus. The two seasons can feel conflicting if the dark half of the year brings about feelings of sadness. However, autumn can bring a lovely balance to the outward energies of inner spring, allowing motivation and passion to expand at a soft, gentle pace. Remember to be gentle with yourself.

Inner spring and yearly winter

If you inwardly tussle with the colder months, your renewed sense of planning and goal-setting may feel dampened. This is something to consider as you move into the shorter days. Give yourself more time to rest and lower your expectations a little, if you need to. You may also find that winter allows your inner spring to manifest and build visions from a more "dreamy" place. The dark, sacred days of winter nurture goals from a spiritual and reflective perspective.

 ## Spring and the life cycle

We can also look at our inner seasons through the prism of our life seasons: Maiden, Mother, Wild Woman and Crone. Attuning to interplay of our menstrual and life seasons helps us listen to the intricate insights and wisdom of our mind, body and spirit. If you find your inner spring season difficult, it may be worth looking at how you currently experience, or did experience, the spring of your life.

Spring and Maiden

A world of possibility and wonder may open at every corner as these two phases match up. You may relish intensified feelings of confidence and enthusiasm, painting the town red and getting all kinds of experimental. It can feel like there's too much to be getting on with and not enough time to get it done! If the Maiden feels any pressure, or inadequacy taking up space, spring may feel disorienting. Pay attention to old perfectionist habits here.

Spring and Mother

As the Mother phase in the life cycle centres on blossoming, you may feel it's easy to lift others with your natural inner spring charm and charisma. Spiritual strength from community healing is also at the heart of this life phase, so you wonder how others experience things and learn a few lovely lessons in the process. A stumbling block is if you're working with the shadow Mother energies of being overly responsible for others. You may not experience a ready sense of playfulness that can optimize this menstrual phase. Here, remember to laugh and look for pockets of light and fun.

Spring and Wild Woman

A fresh spring take on the world, with the Wild Woman confidence can be truly potent. The unrestricted energies of both of these cycles can really amplify any experience, right now. We can also be at our most discerning. What a combination! However, spring may not always feel like a rising energy of new beginnings if we're experiencing peri-menopausal symptoms. As our inner seasons can echo our life seasons, it's also worth looking at whether there's anything you regret, or feel disappointed about, from your younger years that's showing up in your menstrual season of spring.

Spring and Crone

No longer bleeding, you can feel empowered to act on whatever feels good. Both spring and Crone hook into the "beauty of the moment" with a softness that enjoys the route as much as the destination.

As with the yearly season, spring is full of potential and rising excitement. Our self-care sessions help us hold the beautifully opposing strengths of vulnerability and potency while we navigate this time of new beginnings. Optimizing this phase on a mind, body and soul level allows the seeds of possibility to take root. There is much to feel hopeful about as we flow with the surges of positivity and purpose, savouring the path to summer fullness.

CHAPTER 14

INNER SUMMER

Inner summer invites you to take the stage, gorgeous one, and the play is all about you.

The lovely, delicate seeds of inner spring have been nursed and tended to, and now the flower is ready to fruit. What might this look like for some of us? We may feel productive at work, more physically active, creative in our needs, communicative and loving at home, and/or empowered to show up fully in everyday moments.

This phase appears after inner spring, between days 12 and 19 (if you have a 28-day menstrual cycle). During this time, we ovulate (egg gets released) and we tend to feel at our physical best. Emotionally, we're entering outward energies of creativity and pleasure. On a mystical level, we're allowing fullness and aliveness to inhabit our spiritual selves.

Expressing your true power is to be experienced in its entirety here. An energetic version of you blossoms as you enter this shiny, fertile phase. Life can feel easier and more pleasurable. It's a time to give yourself the recognition you need and deserve, rejoicing in a celebration of your beautiful self (without any belittling inner monologue).

And even more mouth-watering – we can do all this while remaining tuned into the needs of others. We tick every box, right now, presenting the version of ourselves that the world wants us to be. For this reason, the inner summer season can feel addictive.

However, inner summer can only be joyful if we fully accept its transience. For our fruit to blossom, our inner spring seedlings need to be treated with sensitivity. We also need to allow autumn to come along. If we push to extend this phase when autumn arrives, we close ourselves off to the darker days and the riches that live there. The brilliance of inner summer is that it is a culmination of each stage.

As with each of the inner seasons, there's not one specific way to experience your summer. For some, this phase isn't bursting with joy. What happens if we don't like what there is to express? If you're not OK with being seen, this season can feel directionless with the heart's pull to hide from the world. If we harbour any shame or self-doubt, these may peak instead of the positive summer traits of desirability and creativity. Because of this, you can feel exposed or overwhelmed.

Our summer self-care sessions that follow can help you to connect with the joyful parts of yourself, learning how to mother yourself, actively and unashamedly.

PHYSICAL HEALING

Much like the vibrancy of the summer months when flowers bloom and fruits are in season, our inner summer is our most fertile time. Even if we're not considering pregnancy, we may feel "fertile" with increased energy and vitality.

You are most fertile during your 20s until your mid-30s and release about 500 eggs throughout your lifetime. Oestrogen reaches a peak just before ovulation. This hormone impacts every part of your body, including the brain, so you will feel more alert and energized. A spike in luteinizing hormone (LH) then occurs, triggering the release of the egg into your fallopian tube midway through your cycle. If this egg is fertilized with sperm within two days, it moves to the uterus over the next week or so (6–12 days) to implant for possible pregnancy. Progesterone is the dominant hormone after ovulation. If the egg isn't fertilized, the corpus luteum (a yellow body that forms in the ovary every cycle) starts to deteriorate, causing a drop in hormones, and consequently your period.

Many factors impact ovulation, including nutrition, feelings and energy. With all this going on, how can we support the body during inner summer?

 ## Nourish yourself

As you may feel more active from the peak of sex hormones at this time, eating protein to support your energy levels is a great move here. Good protein sources can look like beans, lentils, tofu, organic poultry and quinoa. We also need good fats from foods like wild salmon, nuts and seeds to support our bodies.

Foods rich in vitamin E (e.g. almonds, spinach and sunflower seeds) and vitamin B6 (e.g. wild salmon, sweet potatoes and avocados) can help to bring hormones into balance.

The inner summer can be a fantastic time to eat "cooling" foods due to the increase in basal body temperature, so crisp salads and raw veggies are great. Salads and vegetables are also high in antioxidants, which can support your liver to metabolize any excess oestrogen. Raw carrots (skin-on) and broccoli sprouts are good for this.

You may find that, as this is your busy time, you lose your appetite for food (or forget to eat), so stay mindful and top up the fuel tank. And don't forget your magnesium, as this is your ally in every stage of your menstrual cycle. I would recommend a magnesium supplement as well as eating foods rich in magnesium, such as greens, nuts, seeds and bananas.

 ## Vulva low-down

The oestrogen peak and the increased testosterone will mean your body produces more cervical fluid, making this the wettest phase of your menstrual cycle. Your cervical fluid may feel slippery with a stretchy, egg-white consistency. It can help maximize your feelings of pleasure and helps potential sperm fertilize any awaiting egg. Your body feels ready for closer intimacy as your sex drive increases and it prepares for possible pregnancy. This is the optimum time to have sex if you're looking to conceive (and to be extra careful if you're not!).

As we transition from inner spring to summer, the cervix climbs higher in the vaginal canal, feeling softer to the touch. You may feel some light cramping in the pelvis during ovulation. As the ovaries usually take turns to ovulate, you will probably feel these tinges on one side one month, and on the other side the next month.

 ## Sex and intimacy

Get ready to roll your sleeves up as now is the time to go for it ... if you want to. This is a great time to go on dates, so embrace that summer lovin', and just remember that you are at your most fertile! But also, please don't put yourself under pressure if you are keen to try for a baby.

During inner summer, we feel tapped into pleasurable senses and in symphony with our needs. If we're flowing with this phase, it can feel deeply sensual. You may want to try a new position or play out any lingering fantasies, either with yourself or with others, as it's likely to be your most turned-on stage.

Communication is also peachy, so ask for what you want in bed. There's no shame in expressing your desires; instead, it will lead to a better relationship with yourself and others. Capitalizing on your shiny, sexy energies is beautiful.

 Skin love

Ovulation-time skin can feel like the holy grail as this is when we're more likely to experience a clear, bright complexion from the peak of oestrogen just before the egg releases. Moisture levels and collagen can make your skin feel and look at its best.

On the flip side, as the hormone levels change in relation to each other, breakouts can occur. When testosterone is up in comparison to other hormones, sebum can go on overdrive, clogging pores. If you're struggling with midway-cycle spots, you're not alone, as ovulation acne affects around 54 per cent of the female population, and it's more likely to show up on the lower half of the face, especially around the mouth, chin, jawline, and also between the eyebrows.

One way to help with this problem is to get rid of excess dead skin cells by using products that contain glycolic or salicylic acid, or fruit enzymes, but only if they don't irritate your skin in any way, so be sure to try a sample first.

Getting good-quality sleep, drinking plenty of water and looking after your gut health also carry their weight in gold when it comes to good skin health, and will help you feel good all month round, more to the point.

 ### Exercise

Syncing your body with the natural rhythms of the inner seasons means you can challenge yourself with higher-intensity workouts this week. If you're the kind of person who wants a new personal best, summer is the optimum time to stretch yourself further.

Oestrogen can respond well to higher-intensity movement. Toward the end of summer, when oestrogen drops off and progesterone takes over, you may want to ease off a little. Make sure to warm up properly, as you might be slightly more susceptible to injury.

There are so many ways to be active. Put on some music and dance around to increase oxygen-rich blood flow to the brain and feel in tune with the sensual summer energy of this phase. And if you're lucky to live somewhere near nature, taking regular long walks to connect with Mother Earth can be a great way to keep your body healthy.

If you're hoping to conceive, any exercise that increases blood flow to the pelvis is great now. Yoga inversions (such as on page 126) or any pose that brings your hips higher than your heart helps carry sex hormones from the brain to the rest of your body.

GODDESS YOGA POSE

Unleash your power with this yoga pose, which releases fear and welcomes your full potency to circulate. This position also helps to strengthen the lower body, stimulate the pelvis and connect you to your pleasure-seeking energies, reminding you that you're worthy of feeling deep-body joy.

1. Stand with your feet wide apart. Lift your arms out to the sides at shoulder height and bend your elbows until your lower arms are at 90° to your upper arms. Turn your palms out or toward you, depending on what's most comfortable.
2. Turn your feet out so y̶ ̶ ̶ ̶ ̶f̶a̶c̶i̶n̶g̶ ̶a̶w̶a̶y̶ from you.
3. Exhale and bend your k   ur ankles. Look straight ah   your pelvis tucked in as muc   ur back long and straight.
4. Hold the pose for thre   n your capability. To release, i   our legs. Gently bring you

 Sleep on it

The heavy dose of summer steamy thoughts, plus the change in body temperature, can lead to sleep difficulties at ovulation. Basal body temperature drops leading up to the release of the egg and increases after. If you are burning up (literally, as well as metaphorically), you might find it trickier to drop off a night. If this is you, here are three quick hacks to help:

1. Wind down a good hour before bedtime – this means turning off screens.
2. Have a warm bath before bedtime – the body losing heat afterwards is the thing that helps you get to sleep.
3. Sleep in lighter bed clothes and bedding, especially just after ovulation when the basal body temperature increases.

EMOTIONAL HEALING

And let there be love. During inner summer, expansive energies can help us connect to both our inner and outer world. However, inner summer can also feel emotionally exhausting if we're giving away too much to others and hiding too much of ourselves.

 Curiosity writing prompts

These reflective questions can deepen self-awareness and offer direction when this outwardly focused phase feels off-balance. Journalling unloads all that summer mind chatter onto paper, giving us those all-important "aha" moments.

- When do you feel most alive?
- When do you feel most flat?
- If you were to introduce yourself to a friend, what lovely things would you say?
- Which people in your life feel like the sun and who takes too much from you?
- What plans are you most looking forward to?
- What here-and-now pleasures do you sink into?

- If your body could speak, what would it say and what does it need?
- Is there anything that stops you from believing that you're enough?
- How do you feel about the idea of being seen?
- How do you feel when you're not coping, or being seen as not coping?
- How are you taking care of yourself during the other phases of your cycle?
- Where do you see yourself in five years?

 Breathwork: energy flow

Which breathing practice you want to take part in depends on how you want to feel at the end of it. If inner summer is too hot, you may want to take it down a notch with some calming breaths. Or if you want to turn up the heat, you can practise some breath boosters. Your answer will dictate which breathwork practice is best for you.

TURN IT UP: DOUBLE-BREATHING

This will help you feel more alert and allow in that high energy.

1. Take a breath in through your nose with a short, strong inhalation followed by a longer, strong inhale in that same breath.

2. Breathe out through your nose with a short exhale, followed by a longer exhale.
3. Repeat this four to seven times depending on where you are with your breathwork journey.

TURN IT DOWN: 4–7–8 BREATHING

This will help you reduce ovulation jitters, improve sleep and lower your blood pressure by activating the parasympathetic nervous system.

1. Breathe in through your nose for the count of four beats.
2. Gently pause at the top of the breath for seven beats.
3. Breathe out through your nose for the count of eight beats.
4. Repeat this four to seven times depending on where you are in your breathwork journey.

 ## Mindful eating

Get ready to savour the moment with a mindfulness eating exercise. This can help you connect to juicy summer energies and the beauty of your food.

1. Choose a ripe piece of fruit and take a bite.
2. Absorb the experience, noticing the taste, texture and smell. How does it feel?

3. Enjoy the ritual of eating and paying full attention to the experience without the distraction of screens or your ever-demanding to-do list.

4. Consider the steps your food went through before you could eat it and take a moment to acknowledge that it's your beautiful source of life.

 ## Loving kindness meditation

Meditation is so beneficial for us during inner summer as it helps us focus on the moment and feel more creative. Here's the chance to enhance our summer energy and slow down the need to overdo things. We need to be present with our hearts and the fullness of self-love to feel fully aligned with this season.

1. Bring yourself to a comfortable position – sitting with a straight spine is great. If you want to lie down, this works absolutely fine here, too.

2. Place your hands on your heart centre, at the middle of your chest. This is where emotions enter.

3. Gently stay with your heart, allowing your breath to flow into this centre. Whatever you feel, or whatever your heart says, it's perfect. There is no right or wrong here. Understanding the wishes of your heart allows the flow of love.

4. Just be with your heart for as long as you need. When the time feels right, gently nudge yourself out of the meditation by bringing your awareness back to the room you're in and gently flutter your eyes open.

Big conversations and empathy in relationships

Hello, tolerance! The things we may find irritating during our inner autumn can feel endearing during our inner summer. It may be worth giving your significant other a heads-up that you're in the love zone. Next week, things may look *quite* different! And that's just it; you will be a different person each week over the month, and that's OK.

As you're likely to empathize with others more easily during your inner summer, having bigger conversations can feel easier. If there's something that's been niggling away for some time, your midway point is a great moment to have a conversation you've been avoiding. You're more likely to be more open-minded, expressive in your needs or expectations, and able to step into the other person's shoes.

Peak communication skills mean if you want something, whether that's at work or home, ask for it. Be it a promotion at work or asking your partner (or parent) for something you want them to say "yes" to, you're more likely to get it over the line in this menstrual phase. If you find communication tricky in this phase, try leaving your loved one a note. Lovingly explaining your challenges and what you need them to see through the written word, can be a less intimidating way of expressing your needs.

If you are a parent, this is the optimum time to play, chat, help your child or teenager in whatever they need, and explain inappropriate behaviour from a calm place. Being "in service" during this phase can feel lovely. Whether that's getting someone's shopping in, listening to a friend in need or cooking a meal for someone, this is prime "giving out" energy time.

You might feel more sociable than usual, so if you've got an invitation to go somewhere, why not accept it? This is a great time to schedule some overdue shindigs. The best part of this summer phase is that you will have more energy to stay out a little later.

When the inner autumn enters our space, we'll need healthy boundaries, drawing on the art of saying "no". Saying "yes" in summer is good ... as long as it feels good. Remember to be mindful of your needs and only give as much as is right for you.

SELF-LOVE: BODY MASSAGE

Time to revel in your goddess self with some sensual self-touch. This is a dynamic way to free up our deeply sensual selves, moving away from male gratification or patriarchal disapproval. You can skip this massage if it doesn't feel right, although it's always worth wondering why.

You will need:
- plain coconut oil or an oil or cream that you know feels good for your skin

1. When it feels right and comfortable, simply "drop down" into your body for a while by finding a warm, quiet space, putting on some relaxing music and simply "being" with yourself.
2. Apply some oil to your hands, and connect with yourself by moving your hands over your skin. Appreciate your divine self and the many ways it serves you.

3. Feel deserving of these pockets of self-love. You might feel the need to comfort or hug yourself. Or you might want to explore your more erotic side and self-pleasure.
4. If negative thoughts pop into your head, come back to your breath. Breathe slowly in and out through your nose, noticing the pause at the end of the inhale and exhale.
5. Gently come back to your outside world when you're ready.

SPIRITUAL HEALING

We are life givers, and this doesn't relate to whether we can, or choose, to have children. Life-giving relates to the potent and creative feminine life force that breathes unwavering wisdom into our everyday moments. Some of us might feel quite lightheaded on the ovulation nectar of the summer phase.

Paradoxically, fitting in with a templated version of "acceptably sociable" womanhood can feel "too nice". If showing up to the world feels like a fearful place, summer can be a difficult phase.

Looking at this phase through the lens of mysticality, we invite spiritual growth and a manifestation of our truth without the urgency to be "more than", and by this, I mean anything that doesn't look like self-acceptance.

FOLKTALE STORY: ÁINE

Áine, pronounced "awn-ya", is recognized as a fairy queen, known for her healing remedies and good luck magic. She was honoured as the giver of abundance. Farmers would pace their fields on the summer solstice, straw torches in hand, and the wish for protection and prosperity in their hearts.

Celebrated as a natural healer, Áine healed the sick on All Heal Night and sang comforting melodies to the dying in the light of the full moon, facilitating their journey to the Otherworld. She could bring deserving ears creativity and inspiration, or drive someone to madness with the sound of her harp.

Unrestrained, Áine would enjoy different lovers, bearing many Faerie-human children and teaching women about their divine sexuality. But she is not to be crossed. One story tells us how she bites the ear of the King of Munster, Ailill Aulom, when he sexually assaults her, stripping him of his sovereign powers.

Are you getting a many-sided impression of Áine yet? Áine highlights the duality of each phase and the forked aspects of summer. Two things can be entirely true at the same time. This summer folklore tale gives us the framework to understand our natural paradoxes.

Goddess of the earth and the lake, the moon and the sun, love and wrath, Áine asks us to sit with our shadow and our light, knowing every face of our unique worldliness. In this immersive experience, we can honour our truest cyclicality and the essence of unapologetic womanhood.

Self-expression: everyday sensuality

Sensual expression vibrates in many ways, in the bedroom and otherwise. Pleasure can be communicated in our everyday waking moments. Little pockets of ecstasy exist right on our doorstep – we just need to know how to stop and notice them. Learning to breathe sensuality into the "same old" of our daily routines re-ignites our passion for everyday life. It's not what you do, it's how you do it, and life can be a sensual exploration of the little things that make you feel alive.

1. Start by allowing moments into your being as though nothing else counts. Some ideas for you are:

   - Notice the warmth of the shower on your skin.
   - Listen to the rustling of leaves when you walk to work.
   - Sing along to your favourite song as you wash up.
   - Enjoy the simplicity of taking a full, deep breath.
   - Notice the sound of your friend's voice on their voice note.
   - Notice your child's wonderful smile.
   - Observe the phase of the moon.

2. Slow down to a place of complete presence in these moments, noticing how all your senses react when you sink into this fullness.
3. Acknowledge that this moment is just for you. How you arrive at this moment expresses how you show up to life. Sink in with deep pleasure.

Crystals: contentment

Whether you already have a witch's collection of crystals or are simply crystal curious, these stones can be a little portal of power, helping you magnify your spiritual potency.

A lovely crystal to work with for inner summer is rose quartz. Lifting you off your feet with a bear hug, this gem enriches self-love, inner healing and feelings of contentment. Its soft, harmonious feel can help with the shadow side of summer, inviting you to walk through life at a more tender and connected pace.

Rose quartz is thought to aid jealousy, fertility, unworthiness and relationship co-dependency with its vibrations of the Mother archetype. Try wearing your crystals to romanticize sacred little things in the summer phase, or meditate with it by holding it close to your chest and focus on a loving energy entering your heart space.

 ## Womb ritual: sacral chakra

This inner summer ritual can help shed stagnant energy and bring your spring seeds of intentions (see page 48) to life. This is even more fulfilling when done in the sun. Your sacral chakra is located around your womb space, just below your navel.

1. Find a comfortable spot in nature, or, if this isn't possible, in the comfort of your garden or home.
2. Start breathing fully into your womb space, just below the navel. With each inhale, breathe in the beauty of nature, taking in the sun's energy of joy and life.

3. Imagine, as you breathe, this area filling up with a swirling orange glow, a vortex of power that creates more energy with each breath.

4. As you exhale, imagine letting go of anything that no longer serves you. As you inhale, imagine feelings of bliss and pleasure soaking into your sacral chakra.

5. In your mind's eye, imagine yourself giving birth to your seeds of intentions. What does it feel like? What can you see? Make this image as clear and real as possible – as though this is actually happening.

6. When you're ready, bring yourself back to the space you're in with a renewed sense of magnificent possibility.

 ## Summer affirmations

Use these summer affirmations to bring you focus and optimize your spiritual health. You may like to say them in the mirror, use them during a meditation, or write them as notes to put up around your home as a reminder of what a powerhouse you are.

I am worthy of sexual expression.
My womb is a sacred space.
I connect to the fullness of myself and nurture this in others.
I let go of the need to overprotect myself and others.
I am strong and soft, boundaried and loving.
I stay rooted in my path for the highest good.
I am the fullness of the sun and moon.
I am deserving of self-love.

Essential oil: geranium

Geranium is our summer celebrity with its hormone-balancing properties. This uplifting and inspiring essential oil can connect you to that inner summer creativity, but also can gently relax and ground you, preventing those ovulatory highs from toppling over.

Geranium can also help us connect with the loving energies of our heart chakra, balance our mood, relieve tension and reduce symptoms of menopause. You can apply geranium oil mixed with a carrier oil to the wrist, or burn in a diffuser to offer a lovely sense of fullness.

 ## Cosmic ceremony: mothering

A sense of belonging felt within a group of remedying women is soul-restoring. When you're in the inner summer zone, getting together with others feels at its most appealing. As with the other seasons, homing in on a theme can bring commitment and focus to the gathering.

Of course, you may be in the inner summer but your community might not be. So, get to know where each of you are, and what might be a good topic to talk about to bring you all together. It could be anything that feels right, whether self-care, boundaries, inner child work, body love, how to look after our planet, how to connect to sensuality, how to be deeply inclusive of others or even a goddess that is of interest.

A ritual with an inner summer theme is "Mothering". This can be a theme for every season, as many of us live with Mother wounds (see page 18). Focus on how to mother ourselves and how to mother each other. In your group, share what it means to feel truly mothered in life.

Ask yourself questions, such as:

- *What are your inner child's strengths?*
- *What does your inner child need right now?*
- *What kind of words can I say to my inner child?*
- *How can we truly see and hear each other as a community of women?*

If any of these questions are triggering, it may be worth coming at this from more of a general perspective: we are here for each other and really see each other.

When you have shared, it can be a cleansing practice to take turns to look at each other, one by one, in the eyes and say: "You belong. You matter. You are loved".

INNER SUMMER AND OTHER CYCLES

Your inner summer experience may be swayed by the moon, seasons and life cycles. So let's journey into how your inner seasons can be impacted by these three other ways of living cyclically.

 Summer and the lunar cycle

Weaving lunar insights into your menstrual cycle journey can help you make sense of your inner world more intricately. Seeing ourselves more clearly deepens awareness and allows us to flow more easily through life. How may your menstrual summer feel according to the phases of the moon?

Summer and the new moon

Here you are said to be on a "red moon" cycle, indicating a journey of inner development, self-actualization and coming to power. As a result, you may be working on some shadow-self elements. It's thought that the red moon cycle is associated with the high priestess or wise woman. This can mean a more creative expression of yourself and your spiritual needs. You may find yourself paving the way for others, naturally enriching them with your bursts of intuition and wisdom.

Summer and the waxing moon

If you're ovulating on a waxing moon, you are thought to be on a "purple moon" cycle, representing transition, self-discovery and a desire to glean more meaning from your life. You may feel drawn to looking at certain aspects of your life from a deeper perspective and to use this knowledge to call for change.

Summer and the full moon

If you're ovulating with the full moon, this is called a "white moon" cycle. Full moon ovulation is considered to be the embodiment of the Mother or nurturer archetype. This may mean experiencing a part of your life where your purpose centres around care – caring for yourself and others. If you're a bit run down here, it may mean you're giving away too much and need to nurture *your* self-care.

Spring and the waning moon

If you're ovulating with the waning moon, you're considered to be on a "pink moon" cycle, showing the need for self-discovery. You may feel even more ready to enjoy new experiences and come into your power. If you're struggling with moving out of your comfort zone, this can help you stretch forward and be challenged in the process.

MOON SPELL FOR EMPOWERMENT

By keeping our summer energies alive with a moon spell, we can create an intention of empowerment. This can look slightly different depending on how you're feeling and what lunar phase you find yourself ovulating within. Empowerment can be anything you choose: self-awareness, creativity, abundance, self-care, community, assertiveness ... What's it to be?

You will need:
- candle, the colour of the cycle that you're ovulating within (red, white, pink or purple)
- pinch of ground nutmeg (for luck)
- pinch of ground cinnamon (for personal strength)
- moonstone (or something silver)
- sunstone (or something gold)

1. Light the candle and gently dust the nutmeg and cinnamon onto the flames. It's OK if they crackle a little. As you

sprinkle on the spices, imagine a feeling of empowerment coming alive in your space.

2. Hold the moonstone with your left hand and the sunstone with your right hand.

3. Say the spell out loud:

    "With the strength of my summer and with the energy of the moon, may my wisdom flow through me, allowing me to illuminate my magical power and beauty."

    You can now add a specific intention of empowerment that you would like to bring to your inner or outer world. For example, "I achieve great things at work with positivity, persistence and courage".

4. Watch the flames dance for a while, with a quiet knowing in your heart and a smile on your face. Keep hold of your crystals while you imagine your intention of empowerment becoming more real.

5. When you're ready, safely extinguish the candle and show gratitude for your practice today.

 ## Summer and the yearly cycle

Our inner summer will be more fruitful when we understand how this time of expansion and creativity can shift naturally with the movement of the external seasons. Let's take a closer look at how your inner summer might change throughout the year.

Inner summer and yearly spring

Enjoy the fruits of your inner summer but with a dedication to vulnerability and tenderness. Winter has only just passed so you'll want to get back out into the world, especially when your inner summer is shouting at you, but you must unfurl slowly and experiment with sensitivity. Get rid of any urgency here, otherwise you might rush out on centre stage without knowing your lines properly. Enjoy the outwardly focused energy *but* with a feeling of "dipping your toe in" rather than diving head first.

Inner summer and yearly summer

This could be fireworks! This is a time for expansion and fulfilling your seeds of intention. Check in with yourself regularly so you're walking into the full midday sun with some protection. If you're prone to difficult inner summers, you may want to practise anchoring yourself in your body and work on any fears surrounding showing up in the world. You can anchor yourself by observing nature, meditating, practising yoga, going swimming and getting good-quality sleep.

Inner summer and yearly autumn

Autumn calls us to shed, so you can experience the summer tingles knowing that your yearly cycle is transforming into one of deepened self-awareness. Here, you can be visible to the world with your extra dose of midway hormones, but perhaps with a "this is the real me" energy. Autumn is the home of shadow, so you may want to use your inner summer communication skills with a layer of good boundaries as you'll be tending to things that no longer serve you during this part of the year.

Inner summer and yearly winter

Inner summer and yearly winter contain many paradoxes as this is the inner season of birthing intentions and the outer season of death and transformation. How can we marry the two? Saying "yes" to the world but with an inner knowing and good self-awareness is your starting point. Ask yourself questions like: How is my inner truth guiding my purpose and projects? What are my core values and how does my dedication to these fulfil my direction in life? What can I let go of to make space for?

 ## Summer and the life cycle

If you find your inner summer season tricky, it may be worth looking at how you experience, or experienced, the summer of your life. If this is, or was, a challenging time in your life cycle, you may find parts of your inner summer difficult. A person's inner summer can be a busy time with a mix of added responsibilities. If this is the case, you may find that parts of your life summer and menstrual summer can feel tiring from being pulled in too many directions. Or you may find inner summer to be a potent time of creativity and joy, whatever life season you find yourself in.

Summer and Maiden

As we know, our younger years can be full of excitement and anticipation so combining this with the outward energies of inner summer can mean you're bringing your visions to fruition. Make sure you honour your needs with this cyclical mix. It can be so easy to fall into the trap of proving ourselves to the world in our 20s. Going into each phase "too extra" might mean you unconsciously skip the lovely blessings each one has to offer.

Summer and Mother

Creativity and compassion can flow when it's an all-round summer sensation. You may feel like you're really peaking in life if you're in your 30s, and so can delight in your midway inner summer strengths of charm, positivity, sensuality and deep allowing. The other side of the coin may feel like you're burning out with too much heat, feeling like you're on a conveyor belt of output. If this is the case, calm things down a little, even in micro-doses.

Summer and Wild Woman

You can approach your inner summer with clear eyes and a sense of: "I can be productive but outcomes are not indicative of my worth." On the flip side, if you're struggling to flow with the ageing process, you may have a bittersweet feeling that your inner summer highs are behind you. This creates the opportunity to embody the newer spiritual gifts of the autumn years, which are truly magical.

Spring and Crone

If you're in your post-menopausal or winter years, you are magnificent and wise, and I can teach you nothing. In a society that indoctrinates us to believe that our worth is our youthfulness, we can remember that women grow in beauty, wisdom and intelligence as they grow in years.

The inner summer well is full. Full of power, sensuality, creativity and adventure, we feel every desire to burst into bloom. Deep self-care makes sure we extend into fullness without spilling over the edge. Staying grounded is our North Star as the menstrual seasons shift gears again. The first half of our cycle is for developing and creating; the second half is for learning and retreating. As our busy inner summer closes down for the season, we get ready for the quieter days ahead.

CHAPTER 15

INNER AUTUMN

Oh, hi there, Cruella! Is someone getting on your last available nerve? If so, you're probably in your menstrual autumn.

Much is going on behind the scenes and it's time to dig deeper. This phase appears after inner summer and before inner winter, roughly between days 20 and 27, if you have a 28-day menstrual cycle.

On a physical level, this is our premenstrual or luteal phase and progesterone is the primary sex hormone at play. Emotionally, this is a time to go inward. The autumn strengths of honesty and perception emerge (Hello, bullshit detector ...), but so do the drawbacks of irritability and self-criticism. Spiritually, we're navigating seeing our deepest truth with more transparency.

The shiny inner summer and its appealing characteristics of joyfulness and high energy have taken a bow. Everyone (including you) has enjoyed the delicious fruits, but now it's time to allow a different energy to have its way; one that's not as agreeable to the outside world. Inner autumn has a more intolerant, discerning and truth-speaking framework, and suddenly life can feel hard-going.

In our linear world, we're required to be perpetually busy, but we need time below the surface to nourish our relationship with our deepest selves. The natural order of things asks us to retreat, assess and let go.

Sitting with the vulnerabilities of what you must let go of is a crucial part of this premenstrual phase. Inner autumn allows us to feel more in tune with what no longer serves us, in connection with our personal stories and how other people relate to us.

As autumn leaves descend from the tree, your cycle urges you to fall back a little, saying "no" and turning inwards.

Some unhelpful behaviours will come to the fore in this season, and you're being called to meet them with willingness and self-compassion. And when you do this, you will change and heal a little each time. With autumn's good vision, *your* truth feels closer.

Another upside to this beautiful clear-sightedness is enhanced detail-oriented and analysis skills, supporting your everyday experience. Autumn feels like a good time to run over something at work or home with greater consideration.

Sensory processing and perception skills are elevated with progesterone so you may recall things to memory more easily. Your troubleshooting skills will be on top form, making problem-solving and decisions easier. Unless the inner critic spoils things, that is …

Autumn can also be an absolute horror movie as the inner critic attempts to eclipse autumn's strengths. This season is the usual crash pad for negative self-talk and cynicism, and so many of us find the transition into the luteal phase after ovulation to feel like a real blow to the system.

Autumn is uncomfortable and it's supposed to be, but unless we have the coping strategies and self-care ingredients to know how to deal with self-criticism, it's suffocating. We can feel lost and angry. It's a (valid) rage toward the world for expecting us to jump through hoops when we crave quiet. And it's a resentment toward ourselves for being (falsely) inadequate.

For us to own all sides of ourselves and feel supported in who we are, we need a bedrock of strategies and practices to support our mind, body and soul so that we don't automatically hit the self-destruct button. As the physical, emotional and spiritual are interwoven, we cannot bring ourselves into a place of power without working on all three aspects. The luteal phase really needs some extra scaffolding ... so let's start building.

PHYSICAL HEALING

We start making progesterone just after ovulation, which peaks during our inner autumn, about day 21, and then drops off completely just before menstruation. Progesterone, which is produced by the corpus luteum, takes up the baton of preparing the womb lining so that it can receive a fertilized egg. If pregnancy doesn't take place, the corpus luteum dissolves and progesterone drops, which causes the start of menstruation.

Progesterone really is our leading lady. With her abilities to calm the mind, boost the immune system, lower blood pressure and protect the bones, she plays a vital part in the menstrual cycle and is the dominant sex hormone in the luteal phase.

 Nourish yourself

The peak in progesterone during your inner autumn will mean you need more calories and nutrient-dense meals to make you feel full and satisfied. Protein and complex carbs are your pals!

We need extra protein to fortify the endometrium (womb lining), such as chickpeas, sesame seeds and organic turkey.

Complex carbs in the form of wholemeal rice, sweet potatoes and rye break down in your body slowly, helping you feel fuller for longer and reduce PMS cravings. They're great for your blood sugar levels, which are more sensitive during this time. High-fibre fruits like pears and apples are great in this phase too, especially when it comes to premenstrual constipation.

During the latter end of your luteal phase, when both oestrogen (it has another mini rise) and progesterone tail off, you're likely to feel tired and stressed, so increasing serotonin-rich foods will help stabilize premenstrual mood swings. These can include nuts, seeds, soy, dairy and poultry.

We want to keep our cortisol as low as possible because progesterone does *not* like this stress hormone, so PMS will worsen. I'm not a fan of fasting during autumn as it can raise cortisol (which is naturally higher anyway at this point in your cycle) and subsequently decrease progesterone – something we want to avoid at all costs.

A few luteal hacks for you:

- Don't drink coffee on an empty stomach.
- Reduce water retention and stay hydrated by increasing foods that rebalance electrolytes, such as watercress, melons and avocados.
- Eat magnesium-rich foods like nuts, seeds, bananas and dark chocolate – especially if you're craving sweet stuff. Epsom salts in the bath are great, too.

SEED CYCLING

Seed cycling is eating nutrition-packed seeds at different points in your cycle. You can start on any day you like. Eat one tablespoon of your chosen seed, each day, sprinkled into smoothies, yoghurt or oats, as follows:

Luteal phase (Day 15–28): Eat sunflower and sesame seeds to help with bloating, mood swings, breast tenderness and PMS symptoms. These seeds are high in vitamin E, which can help healthy progesterone levels. They also contain vitamins and fatty acids that support the hormones, keeping them balanced.

Follicular phase (Day 1–14): Eat pumpkin and flaxseeds to help balance and detox oestrogen correctly. These seeds are full of phytoestrogens, which helps improve oestrogen levels, while preventing an excess.

 Vulva low-down

Cervical discharge changes with each inner season. You may notice thicker or denser cervical mucus, with a stickier look or feel to it. You may also see a white discharge just before menstruation, which helps keep the vagina clean and healthy. Things might feel a bit dry in the latter stages of the luteal phase, so definitely avoid any perfumed lotions or potions in the bath that could irritate the vulva.

As we move into inner autumn, your cervix drops a bit and may feel firmer to the touch (tip of your nose-type vibes.) However, if conception has taken place, the cervix will likely remain higher in the vagina.

Sex and intimacy

You might feel sleepier and slower in the luteal phase, so it's an opportunity to hand the hard work over. I think inner autumn has a receiving, rather than giving, energy. Sexual desire is more about you, rather than for any biological urge to procreate. For this reason, it can feel freer and more indulgent. I think in autumn, sex has a wilder, "fuck the system" kinda feel to it … Lots of foreplay is also great if things are a bit dry down below, and it's a good idea to use lube (organic, if possible) if you're considering having penetrative sex.

If you're in flow with your wilder sexual energies, it's a great time to evaluate your sex life as inner autumn allows us to go over things with a bit more detail. Ask yourself, and your partner, what feels good or could change. Just remember to apply a wee bit of tenderness when doing so.

On the flip side, the luteal phase is an absolute no-go zone for some of us. Progesterone may decrease sex drive, so getting sexy may be the last thing on your mind. With external pressure and PMS symptoms weighing heavily in this phase, sex can feel unappealing. Plus, having your cervix stimulated (which, as we know, is low at this point) may make certain kinds of sex uncomfortable. Some of us, however, may enjoy this type of arousal and even experience cervical orgasms. Sex can be a real mixed bag here, so just go with your needs and keep communication open with your partner.

 ## Skin love

Clogged pores and sensitivity may be the nature of the beast here. As progesterone peaks so does sebum production, meaning the skin is more vulnerable to breakouts. You may want to focus on using skincare products that have a calming effect, like lavender or aloe vera.

Niacinamide (or nicotinamide) can help with premenstrual flare-ups, calming and smoothing the skin. There are also LED masks with blue light therapy, which kill off acne-causing bacteria, but they are expensive! If premenstrual acne is something that bothers you, try out a purifying face mask that counteracts congested skin.

It's important to approach skin from a holistic viewpoint. Good gut health, keeping hydrated and stress reduction are always extremely important. What's of greatest importance is that as skin changes from month to month, anyway, we need to work on any critical or perfectionist tendencies, above all.

 Exercise

As we know, we have to keep our cortisol levels in check during inner autumn. We already have a multitude of stresses in our everyday lives, and by taking part in too much aerobic or intense exercise, we can put too much pressure on our beloved bodies. This can then have a knock-on effect on our emotional and spiritual health. Unlike oestrogen, which promotes muscle growth, progesterone has a muscle-relaxing effect, so it's really not the time to exercise too hard.

Exercising too much during this phase means we may unintentionally confuse the brain into signalling a protective response, known as the fight or flight mechanism. Fight or flight hormones, like adrenalin, are released into the bloodstream by the adrenal glands after the amygdala hits the panic button. This helps us stay on high alert. If the brain continues to sense something as dangerous (even though it isn't), cortisol is released into the body, forcing the body to stay pumped up. By adding in a fierce workout on top of everything else – work, family commitments, relationships, money worries and all the rest, we may unintentionally aggravate our cortisol levels. And, as we know, when cortisol goes up, progesterone goes down. As progesterone is a calming hormone, this effect isn't a barrel of laughs for mood levels.

Movement is good, don't get me wrong, but exercising our bodies in alignment with our needs and hormones is even better. This is the time in your menstrual cycle to take it down a notch. Walking, Pilates, yoga and some weights are fine (especially if you're in your peri or post-menopausal years) but not to the point where it's exhausting you.

SPHINX YOGA POSE

Work on your adrenal glands and soothe the nervous system with the sphinx yoga pose. This gentle backbend helps to relax the lower back (especially great after long periods of sitting), and also opens the heart, relieving any stress or irritation.

You will need:
- yoga mat or non-slip floor
- loose, comfortable clothing

1. Lie down on your tummy, with your legs hip-width apart and extended behind you, keeping your toes untucked.

2. Place your elbows directly under your shoulders with your forearms parallel to each other.
3. Gently lift your head and chest off the floor. Drop your shoulder blades down and completely switch off the muscles in your bum and legs.
4. Hold this position for a few relaxed breaths.
5. Now slowly release on an exhale by lowering your chest and head to the mat, turning your head to one side.

Sleep on it

Progesterone has a calming effect on the nervous system. This can mean you feel sleepier than during other seasons of your menstrual cycle. When you can, try to go to bed earlier or catch a few winks in the day, during the luteal phase.

Your ability to drift off to sleep can be negatively impacted if your progesterone levels are low, imbalanced or not running at their optimum level. Remember how progesterone goes low with stress? GABA is a neurotransmitter in your brain that helps improve sleep and decrease anxiety. As progesterone stimulates the brain to produce this chemical messenger, insufficient levels can mean poorer sleep. Plus, core body temperature is also higher at night during the luteal phase, which can result in sleep wakings or an inability to sleep.

My top tip here is to offload all your PMS worries before bed. Give yourself ten minutes to actively "worry", writing down everything that's on your mind and any self-critical thinking. This is called "constructive worry". It can help reduce stress and improve the ability to fall asleep. Once your time is up, take some deep breaths and go about your usual, positive bedtime routine. This can involve taking a bath, listening to relaxing music, reducing screen time and practising meditation.

EMOTIONAL HEALING

Feeling pulled in too many directions during inner autumn can make us feel defensive, depleted and even dissociated if things get too overextended. Self-criticism and accusations can run the show. Let's get to the bottom of it all and see what we can do to improve how you feel.

 Curiosity writing prompts

Inner autumn is a call to go within and work out what's happening, why it's happening and how to feel resourceful. Feel free to journal your thoughts or simply spend some time wondering about your answers.

- What overwhelms you the most?
- What triggers your inner critic?
- Who is irritating you and what do they remind you of?
- How would you like your life to be different?
- What do you need to unlearn?
- How do you feel about saying "no" to others?
- How can you treat yourself with greater tenderness?
- How can you safely lean into anger without affecting others?
- What's stopping you from dropping some of your responsibilities?
- Do you believe in the power of your voice?
- How do you feel about asking for help?

BREATHWORK: LION'S BREATH

We need a healthy outlet for PMS tension and self-critical thinking. Lion's breath is an active breathing practice that can release built-up stress and improve self-expression.

1. Organize yourself into a comfortable seated position, either crossed-legged or kneeling. You can have your eyes closed or have a soft gaze.
2. Inhale through your nose and as you exhale, stick your tongue out toward your chin and breathe out forcefully through your mouth. Make a "ha" noise deep from within when doing so, sounding a bit like a roaring lion.
3. Repeat this eight times or for as long as feels right.
4. Come back to the space you're in and find your natural breath before returning to your day.

 ## Mindfulness: amygdala reset

One amazing way to be mindful during this phase is to go on a long walk in nature, and you can do this in whatever external season you find yourself in. This is especially powerful in the early morning, when there are high levels of healthy blue light, and low levels of UVA or UVB (the sun's harmful rays).

Amygdala activity, which is responsible for the fight or flight response we talked about earlier, decreases after a one-hour walk in nature, so you're less likely to experience the emotional stresses of autumn by doing this.

1. Take yourself off somewhere in nature for an hour (less is still good, if you are time-short), and bring a sense of presence to your walk.
2. Notice and get curious about:

- The sounds you can hear.
- The sensation of your feet on the earth below you.
- The way your arms move beside you.
- The rhythm of your walk.
- The season you're in, and the colours and shapes that go with that.
- The smells you're taking in, and the way they remind you of something or someone.
- How you feel when you walk.

 Finding your voice meditation

Autumn irritation bubbles to the surface when we're subjected to too much daily stress – it's a small wonder that life can feel overbearing in this phase. Being "palatable" to others becomes almost impossible, and we start to wonder why we have to swallow unrealistic demands from others. We no longer want to be the "nice girl" and suddenly realize how many people have access to us.

To root into the potential of autumn, we can listen to our inner voice. When we're closed off, we can't express ourselves openly and directly, so we start feeling stuck, annoyed or detached. When our throat centre is balanced, we can speak truthfully but without reacting volatilely. This is a simple, easy but powerful meditation to help us do this:

- Carve out space to get comfortable. This can be seated with a straight back or a more restorative lying-down pose. Close your eyes when you're ready.
- Gently place your hands high on the chest, on top of one another, so your fingers are lightly touching the base of your neck and collarbone.
- Simply listen to your throat centre, allowing your breath to rise as far as your hands. Whatever your voice has to say, it's valid. Sit with that for a while. What does your voice want you to hear?
- Be with your throat centre for as long as it feels OK. When you're ready, bring your attention back to the space you're in and gently flutter your eyes open.

Conflict resolution in relationships

It's easy to get triggered by your nearest and dearest during inner autumn. Relationships can be tough at times, anyway. Trying to marry up two entirely different lived experiences and ways of doing things is tricky, to say the least, but relationship conflict can act as an opportunity for growth, and is very normal.

Your emotions will be running high during inner autumn, so you may feel your frustration escalating, especially if you're having to "contain" yourself all day at work or with children. During autumn, you will want your special someone to really see and hear you, understanding why you're on edge and what they can do to sweeten the tension. However, they won't be able to read your mind. Here are a few simple ideas to feel grounded when resolving conflict or worries in this phase:

- Arrange to have a conversation about your concerns at an appropriate time, when you both have the right kind of head space. Let your person know which phase of your cycle you're in.
- Avoid using inflammatory language such as, "You always …" and deliver your feedback in a specific way, instead of generalizing.
- Actively listen to your partner by hearing where they're coming from, too. Try to do this without trying to compete for "one-upmanship" or interrupting them. Taking notes or concentrating on your breathing when they're speaking is helpful. If their behaviour or words become unhelpful, you can intervene appropriately.
- Avoid trying to "convince" your partner. Instead, find examples of why you feel this way and what you would like to be different in a straightforward, but compassionate, way.
- Don't be afraid of taking a time-out if things get too much out by saying, "I need to step away for a bit as I'm getting too overwhelmed here".
- Recognize old patterns, especially ones that replicate experiences from childhood, and allow your partner into this self-awareness by saying, for example, "I recognize what I'm doing here, and I think I saw my mum act in this same way".

 Self-love: inner critic

This technique helps you learn more about your inner autumn critic from a point of curiosity. Often, we get swept up in critical premenstrual thoughts, but when we learn to take a step back and listen, we can understand ourselves much better and get to an open-hearted place. You can do this practice in any position that feels comfortable.

- Where is the inner critic in your body?
- What does your inner critic look or sound like?
- Why are they here?
- What are they afraid of?
- What do they want from you?

When you have listened to the answers, observe how you now feel toward this part of you. By spending time acknowledging your inner critic, you're telling them that they're important but they don't need to continue to keep you safe.

It's now your turn to respond. What kinder words would you like to say to your inner critic? When you have spent enough time here, move away from this session with a renewed awareness.

ALL GETTING TOO MUCH?

Premenstrual dysphoria disorder (PMDD) is a more extreme form of PMS that causes difficult symptoms during the luteal phase. Critical thoughts go beyond "normal" and life can feel utterly hopeless for some sufferers. If you're worried you may have PMDD or are concerned about any symptoms, contact your healthcare professional. Some people experience suicidal thoughts during the lead-up to their period. Please call the emergency services or Samaritans on 116 123 if this is the case.

SPIRITUAL HEALING

Deepening our autumnal journey, we can look to rituals, stories and spiritual practices to feel more seen and empowered during this phase, aligning ourselves with a deeper sense of truth.

FOLKTALE STORY: MIS

Overcome with fathomless grief after her powerful father, Dáire Dóidgheal, is brutally slaughtered in battle, Mis tosses herself onto his body, sucking at his wounds, attempting to breathe her own life back into him. Taken by a sea of grief and rage, she becomes half woman, half crow, fleeing into the mountains of Sliabh Mis.

After many years of isolation, a young man named Dubh Ruis gently coaxes this fearsome creature back to her old self (or indeed a new version of herself), by reminding her lovingly of how things were before the "madness" of pain snatched her away. After some time, they returned to court together, spending many happy years there before Dubh Ruis was killed. Instead of losing herself to despair again, she channelled her grief into a beautiful poem.

I first encountered the story when reading *If Women Rose Rooted* (see Further Reading) by Sharon Blackie. In her book, she describes the madness that came upon Mis as "... an extreme form of initiation, a trigger for profound transformation". Symbolizing an utter descent into the wildness, both spiritually and literally, the Irish myth identifies a need many of us feel. I can only describe this as a sort of falling apart under the weight of it all. We can then rise from the depths of this rubble.

For me, Mis embodies many things: A tearing apart of the old self, unexpressed grief and a rage at the outer world. By swooping into her shadow self so wildly and unconditionally, she completely vandalizes rational thought and self-control. Do you ever feel that way? Perhaps Mis represents that urge that many of us feel to reject the restrictions of the external world. The doing and the proving ourselves that are still required during our PMS days can feel so utterly repressive, that it becomes an almost contorted experience.

What can we take from this tale? If we can allow ourselves to spiral down into the parts of ourselves that often we keep so unseen during the autumn's descent into inner truth, we have the opportunity to transform our old belief systems.

Our folktale heroine can only return to her community once she's endured a breaking-down journey – a total surrender. As Sharon Blackie says, "... she must find a way to reclaim a more authentic sense of identity and belonging". Here, the belonging of Mis is felt through a man loving her at her most "unappetizing". Your rediscovery can be experienced in many ways, but what it must involve is a transparency of your deepest truth.

 ## Self-expression: somatic anger

Inner autumn holds a mirror to how we experience anger and how those angry feelings were modelled to us by our primary caregivers. When we feel unsupported in our needs, we can get caged in by this anger.

Autumn calls for us to get close to our deepest selves so that we can see what's happening and transform powerful emotions, such as anger, into a sense of purpose and spiritual growth. Instead of getting hung up on the things that can feel so grating in life, set time aside for this session to release stagnant anger on an energetic level.

1. Start by playing some loud music that makes you feel something.
2. Standing, bounce your feet a little on the ground beneath you.
3. Allow this movement to spread higher, shaking both legs and releasing any pressure.
4. Allow this rising energy to spread into your torso, arms and hands, feeling all the feels now.
5. Meet fully whatever comes up for you and let it be free. Really shake off any locked-in energy from all areas of your body, wherever that might be. Feel free to use your voice to release anything unwanted as well. Go wild!
6. When you're ready (and if you need a rough guide, 5–10 minutes works well), start to slow down your movements and return to a standing position.
7. You may need to rest or journal a little after this practice.

 ## Crystals: balance

Stones can enrich your spiritual relationship with inner autumn, and agate is a standout crystal for this menstrual phase. Autumn has a yin energy, which means feminine, inward and slower. Unfortunately, the world wants us to be in perpetual yang, which symbolizes masculine, outward and energetic. Agate can bring the yin and yang energies into balance, stabilizing us into a more grounded and spiritually powerful place. It also helps heal anger and can give us the faith needed to transform the old.

Try keeping your agate crystal somewhere that's busy, like your workspace or in the kitchen to help ward off any negative energies and keep you focussed and grounded in your power, even when there's far too much noise around you.

 Womb ritual: womb grid

Womb grids can be a symbolic way to help self-expression through colours, crystals, flowers, stones and anything else you're attracted to. Creating a womb grid is an intuitive practice that doesn't need any specific skill set.

1. Collect and look closely at some things that you are drawn to; this can be anything from your crystal collection, some plants or flowers collected from the garden, or ethically sourced stones.
2. Breathe deeply and slowly and focus on the feelings around your womb centre. This is energetically known as our "dwelling place".
3. How does it feel? Where feels tight? What does it need? Notice any images and visions that come to mind as you start to imagine your womb grid.
4. Create your grid, which is often a circle (but doesn't have to be) with your collected pieces. You can begin in the centre and move out or start with the outer layer and work your way toward the centre.
5. Gaze at your grid and wonder what your womb grid is telling you and how it relates to your needs.
6. You can move the grid to somewhere special like your altar or a sacred space in your home.

Autumn affirmations

Affirmations are like a loving but firm friend, who can help you meet your deepest self and direct your energy toward spiritual fulfilment. You can say them during meditation, on the bus to work, during your lunch break or any time that suits you, to affirm your autumnal needs.

> *This phase is hard but I have what it takes.*
> *I'm working to own all sides of myself.*
> *I'm as worthy as the earth I walk on and belong here.*
> *To flourish, I create space to rest and retreat.*
> *At times, I say "no" to take care of myself, and those who love me understand.*
> *I heal by speaking my truth.*
> *It's OK to feel uncertain or overwhelmed; I have nothing to prove.*
> *I acknowledge my unique cleverness and intuition.*
> *I trust the process of letting go, surrendering what no longer serves me.*

 ## Essential oil: lavender

Aromatherapy can reduce PMS symptoms and also support our spiritual work. Lavender is beautiful and versatile during inner autumn; it's calming, so can help optimize those luteal analysis skills without the usual overthinking, and it contains truth-speaking and communication properties. Lavender can also help us to sleep better – something many of us need during inner autumn when stress levels are higher.

Bringing the higher and lower chakras into harmony, lavender can also generate an energetic balance on a soul level, allowing greater ease and intuition to flow within us. Try a few drops of essential oil on your pillowcase before you go to sleep or apply topically to your wrist in the morning. You may need to dilute lavender in a carrier oil, such as sweet almond, depending on your sensitivity.

 ## Cosmic ceremony: comparison

Autumn is the home of comparison. When we don't feel good enough, we instinctively look at others to check how we're matching up, perhaps spending too much time on social media. Social comparison isn't new; it is deep-seated in human behaviour. In modern-day life, there are ever more opportunities to feel the grip of benchmarking with the amplification of unrealistic standards, set by social media.

You are not alone in any feelings of perceived failure or powerlessness. Everyone has an inner critic and even the most "successful" folk thought (or still think) they were not good enough. So, what can we do to feel better about ourselves and feel confident in our truth?

Coming together in a ritual of togetherness with your main ladies can help nourish a sense of belonging and lessen comparison. Holding space for one another can chip away at comparison culture and help us feel valued for our unique offering to the world. In your group, set up a sacred space in whatever way feels right. Ask yourself questions, such as:

- Why do we need to be everything to everyone, and how can life look different?
- What comparisons feel triggering and why?

- How can I feel powerful in my own unique experience, and how do I align myself with a sense of purpose?
- How can I pull back and still feel like I'm enough?

When you all have listened and spoken, it can be an affirming practice to take turns to look at each other, one by one, in the eyes and say something like, "The world wouldn't be the same without you".

INNER AUTUMN AND THE OTHER CYCLES

As we now know, the inner autumn experience may be impacted by our other cyclical teachers. Let's venture into how your menstrual seasons can be impacted by the lunar, life and seasonal cycles.

 ### Autumn and the lunar cycle

How can your inner autumn change according to the phases of the moon cycle? Now we have a handle on the inner workings of autumn, we can take this cyclical awareness further by noticing any subtle differences the moon phases may bring.

Autumn and the new moon

Inner autumn and the new moon have a quieter energy, so they pair up quite nicely. However, if you're prone to heavy PMS symptoms, the darkness of the moon can feel like an intense place to be. Honouring your need to go inwards is a wonderful practice during inner autumn, but try not to let it slip into full "lone wolf" (even if that's your bag), as it may cause you to start to wallow in self-critical thinking and miss out on the potency of the new moon. Using inner autumn surrender to clear the way for new moon possibilities may be the ticket here.

Autumn and the waxing moon

So, how do you take action on the goals you have been preparing for during your waxing lunar practices *and* withdraw from the outside world during your autumn menstrual phase? One way is to allow your waxing moon intentions to gently expand with the inner autumnal qualities of clear-sightedness and appraisal. You can really see what needs to happen in your life to move forward from an informed and sharp perspective. Remember to take it easy on yourself; your inner pace will be slower and gentler.

Autumn and the full moon

Things can go one or two ways. The full moon can help pull everything to the top that needs to be seen and healed during your inner autumn, which can feel like a pivotal time in your spiritual journey. Or, you may feel overwhelmed with this potential baptism of fire. You can use this lunar phase to your advantage by coming face to face with those old patterns getting in the way of personal growth, but please do so with your self-care practices to keep your nervous system regulated. Your mind and body will then feel more prepared for the deep energetic shifts. And, as always, reach out for help if things ever feel out of hand.

Autumn and the waning moon

Hello, hermit! This can work deliciously as you are being compelled to simply "sit in the void". Fully and compassionately attending to all sides of yourself means you'll be in a better-equipped place to let go of old patterns. However, the mix of these two phases can feel a little "too close", especially if you have more severe PMS symptoms. Imposter syndrome driven by not feeling deserving can come into the scene at this point. Give yourself a break and root into practices that keep your cortisol low, such as given on pages 73, 74 and 184.

MOON SPELL FOR OVERWHELM

Maintaining grounded autumn energies with a lunar spell can help us set an intention of balance while navigating this challenging and sometimes overwhelming phase. You can do this during any moon phase as the intention here is to simply stay rooted in the present, but now is the perfect time to try this.

You will need:
- mud (see step 1 overleaf)
- dried basil leaves
- bowl
- wooden spoon or stick
- dish to burn a candle in
- brown candle
- matches or lighter

1. Take your shoes and socks off, go outside and collect a handful of mud. By going outside and planting your bare feet onto the grass or into the soil, you discharge any negativity and instantly feel grounded. Dig your hands into the soil and scoop up a little earth ready for your spell.
2. Mix your mud in a bowl with your dried basil leaves (which symbolize clarity and groundedness).
3. Place some of your mixture around the edges of the dish and put your candle in the centre. Next, burn your candle. Imagine your body roots down into the ground beneath you as you watch the candle melt.
4. Say out loud the spell:

   "I anchor myself in the power of the here and now. With the knowledge that I'm as worthy as the earth and as potent as the moon, I am grateful for every single moment."

5. When you're ready, extinguish the candle and go about your day with a renewed sense of centredness.

Autumn and the yearly cycle

Let's take a closer look at how your inner autumn may feel a little differently throughout the seasonal year. The more you understand your cyclical layers, the better you will understand yourself and your needs throughout the months ahead.

Inner autumn and yearly spring

If you're in your inner autumn and it's the external season of spring, you may find this week feels a little lighter than it does in the colder seasons. You may be able to approach those die-hard habits with a sense of achievability now. The luteal challenge of facing yourself can feel easier with the spring gifts of curiosity and possibility. If you prefer, you may want to leave any concrete yearly spring goal-setting for a week or two until you're in the first half of your menstrual cycle.

Inner autumn and yearly summer

Summer calls for self-appreciation; something that doesn't necessarily yoke with inner autumn. The way to get around this is to focus on fulfilment through the lens of being fully present and honest with yourself. Being authentically you by making room for both the light and the shadow can give rise to a total fullness that the external summer season will really appreciate.

Inner autumn and yearly autumn

How you feel about this time depends on how you tend to yourself during autumn: both throughout the month and the year. Falling back from the outer world and finding those moments of retreat can allow for a full-bodied autumnal experience. If things feel murkier, you may find that your inner autumn clashes with its reciprocal external season. Shadow work can feel intimidating. If so, only ever do what you can, and focus on the strengths of good boundaries, remembering to say "no" to anything that requires more than you have to offer.

Inner autumn and yearly winter

Winter has a vulnerability to it. When we enter the week leading up to our period, we may find it even more difficult to shield ourselves from criticisms. To navigate this as best as possible, it's important to see the strengths in being vulnerable while actively nourishing those powerful inner autumn characteristics of intuition and sharpness. You may also find that the slower energies complement each other nicely.

 ## Autumn and the life cycle

The autumnal strengths of self-awareness and intuition can feel even more powerful when we understand this menstrual season in the context of our life cycles. If you find your inner autumn season difficult, it may be worth looking at how you experience the autumn of your life. There will be many of you reading this who aren't there yet, so just go with your life phase.

Autumn and Maiden

The sense of possibility felt during the Maiden years can soften the voice of the autumn inner critic. But if you're finding your 20s feel like a pressure cooker of milestones and comparison culture, your inner autumn can feel a particularly unsympathetic place to be. What's key here is to develop a great sense of self-awareness by tracking your cycling journey. This can help you watch out for any autumn disasters and give yourself some slack.

Autumn and Mother

This life phase is often one of creativity and nurture, so how can we balance this energetic outpouring with the autumnal experience of saying no to the outside world? It comes down to really zeroing in on the capacity for self-love and kindness, as well as being there for others. This will help when it comes to transforming any looming self-criticism into a feeling of unconditional love; something the Mother is so mindful and supportive of.

Autumn and Wild Woman

The combination of perimenopause and PMT can be a hormonal nightmare that hits the mind, body and soul hard. We've got to get our cortisol down as the first port of call. Once the body is on board, we can begin looking into these corresponding seasons with more nuance as there is much power here. Questioning what suits us and awakening to our deepest truth can materialize so robustly with this combination. Others may not like it, however. The premenstrual phase felt during the Wild Woman years can be one of the most significant and revelatory cyclical experiences.

Autumn and Crone

The menstrual journey has come to an end and you have the power to intuit and manifest beyond the power of the inner seasons. There is so much wisdom and consciousness to be discovered during this life phase that doesn't rely on the ebb and flow of inner cyclicality.

Inner autumn shows us the hurt to heal and the skills to sharpen. It's a revelatory week that asks you to become tender with every unique aspect of your being, even the parts you turn away from. Meeting your shadow-self with deep acceptance means you look past the usual limits of the premenstrual days, feeling empowered by the lessons of this season. With each passing autumn, it becomes more natural to retreat back home to yourself, knowing that winter is ready to repair and restore your heart and soul with its nourishing rest.

CHAPTER 16

INNER WINTER

A red tent awaits, goddess.

Inner winter is the time of menstruation, from around day 28 if you have a 28-day menstrual cycle. The day before your period starts marks the onset of inner winter. The last day of your period carries a sense of renewal and clarity that blossoms as you gently remerge into inner spring once more.

Physically, emotionally and spiritually, this inner season is a time of shedding. Hormones die down, signalling to our bodies that it's time to release the endometrium lining. Emotionally, we're invited to drop the schedule and let go a little. Spiritually, it's a simple retreat into the sweetness of existence. Heaven. And yet, it can be a challenging time for some of us.

How do you feel about your period? Is it something you haven't paid much attention to, or is it an inconvenience? Do you dread it because of a menstrual health condition or do you relish this time to be quieter?

The "taboo" of periods, alongside the misunderstandings of female hormonal patterns, makes retreating from the outside world during menstruation intimidating and challenging. How can we withdraw when our commitments demand otherwise? And how easy it is to say, "I need to be at home/do less because I'm on my period". Not very.

Despite menstrual leave being introduced in certain countries and more people opening up about their cyclic experiences, women do not have access to the 24-hour clock that many men work from. A man's hormonal pattern means they can be consistent and efficient daily, which is so very convenient for capitalism. Women slip into a different power during menstruation; one that's far more illuminating than "performance". The problem is these menstrual strengths don't make money or tick an obvious box. Our gifts are presence and worthiness.

Inner winter is our natural urge to cut short the race we can't seem to stop running. It's a realization that we're worthy whether we get to the finish line or not. A power struggle emerges as we're being called to let go and relax, but society seems to demand that we keep at it, for fear of being unsuccessful (and risking the potential of rejection). Unless we appreciate our fallow periods, we risk burnout. We're not cut out for the usual commotion of life at this point. It's not playing into any menstrual tropes that we're under the control of our hormones; it's simply that we ebb and flow throughout the month, and it's OK to know where our power lies this week.

There is an enormous strength in dropping down like the winter tree that sits in the simplicity of nothing. In this nothing, we arrive at real life with a divine authenticity that calls us to gaze beyond the need for more. Your cycle asks you to slip deeper into the ordinary and the small things within and around you. Turning our back on demands is challenging, but without this monthly rite of passage, the well remains dry.

Filling our cup, the sessions in this chapter invite you to appreciate "the slow", helping your mind, body and soul feel nourished and restored.

PHYSICAL HEALING

With an average of 480 periods across a woman's lifetime and each one lasting between three and seven days, it's hardly surprising they're a big bloody deal.

What's happening on a hormonal level? Progesterone plummets when the egg made at ovulation doesn't get fertilized, letting our body know that it's time to release the womb lining. This flow comes out of the uterus through the cervix and consists of blood, cells, tissue and prostaglandins.

Prostaglandins are hormone-like substances that help stimulate muscle contractions in the uterus. If there's too much inflammation in the body, there can be higher numbers of prostaglandins. When this is the case, period pain can be extremely painful. With over 90 per cent of us experiencing menstrual pain and over half of us suffering from dysmenorrhea (severe cramps), reducing inflammation in the body is so key to our wellbeing at this time.

 Nourish yourself

What do you want to eat when it's cold outside? Stews, soups and curries are where it's at. Eating for your inner winter as you would for your yearly winter with wholesome, warming foods containing lots of veggies and spices (ginger and turmeric, especially!) will make you feel toasty on the inside and reduce inflammation in the body.

Magnesium is a must during inner winter due to its potent anti-inflammatory benefits, so remember to top up on seeds, nuts, avocados, kale and dark chocolate. I personally supplement with magnesium glycinate to help reduce my period pain. I also take ibuprofen!

Omega 3s also reduce period pain, so eat plenty of seeds and oily fish (organic and ethically sourced, if possible) in this phase. And I hate to be annoying but the very best way to reduce inflammation in the body is to significantly reduce, or cut out alcohol, sugar and ultra-processed foods.

SUPPORT YOUR GUT

When too many prostaglandins are produced, these chemicals can enter the bloodstream, affecting the gastrointestinal tract. The bowels, as well as the uterus, contract, resulting in more trips to the loo. Food often moves along faster than usual causing diarrhoea-type stools. Keeping your prostaglandins at a healthy level with good nutrition is a great way to help lessen any gut issues in this phase.

As we bleed, we will be shedding iron and minerals, potentially causing low energy. If you have a particularly heavy bleed, you may want to supplement with iron, but always check with your doctor if it is safe for you to do so. Incorporating iron-rich foods, such as dark leafy vegetables or organic beef can help replenish iron levels during menstruation. Vitamin C helps you to absorb iron, so increasing your fruit and veg is amazing too.

I recommend Le'Nise Brothers' *You Can Have a Better Period* when it comes to more specific nutritional advice about menstrual health conditions, such as endometriosis, dysmenorrhea and irregular menstruation.

Some women experience "period flu" at this point. Period flu isn't a virus but carries similar (and sometimes debilitating) symptoms, such as a low-grade fever, headaches and muscle pain. It can happen just before or during someone's period and may be due to the body's reaction to the drop in progesterone. If you're feeling poorly, don't push your body to do anything it doesn't want to, and always seek advice from your doctor if something doesn't feel right.

 ## Vulva low-down

Blood flow is often heavier during the first two days of your period. You probably release about 20–90ml/1–3fl oz of blood (about one or two shot glasses) in total. For some women with very heavy bleeds, it will be more than this. Large clots should always be checked out by your doctor.

ECO-FRIENDLY CHOICES

I'm a big fan of period pants or reusable pads when bleeding. Not only are they cost-effective and eco-friendly, but they don't contain bleach, pesticide residue or fragrances that some sanitary towel and tampon brands do. Keeping away from any synthetic chemicals that can affect our hormones, in general, is a great move.

Checking out the colour of your blood is a great indicator of period health. If that makes you feel "ick", think about why that might be and what you've been taught about periods. Blood that is bright crimson red is usually a good sign of a healthy flow. If you notice brown blood at the beginning or end of your period, it could mean not all the blood was released from the uterus from the last cycle, and it has oxidized. If the blood is grey or orange at any stage, please see your doctor as you may have an infection.

Finally, incontinence symptoms can also worsen during your period, especially if you've had a baby. This is partly due to low oestrogen levels, which changes abdominal pressure. I recommend seeing a women's health physiotherapist if you're experiencing any pelvic floor-related issues on which you could do with specific guidance or advice.

 ## Sex and intimacy

How do you feel about period sex? There are some physical benefits to having intercourse during your bleed; the oxytocin (our love hormone) that women release during sex can help relieve any pain, and the extra blood flow may increase sensitivity in the vagina and vulva. This can make period sex a sensual, loving and enjoyable experience.

If you're in a relationship, how does your partner feel about period sex? Periods are still taboo for many, so it's not surprising that some couples find the whole thing awkward or embarrassing to talk about. Coming from a point of curiosity here can be helpful. Wondering how your partner feels about periods can be a good way to start up an open-minded conversation.

It's possible to still get pregnant during period sex, especially if you're at the very end of your period and have a shorter cycle, as sperm can live in the body for a few days, so be extra cautious if you're not looking to conceive.

If you were hoping to conceive this month, getting your period can be a heart-breaking time, so you may need some space to grieve. There is no right or wrong response here. If you would like to know more about fertility specifically, I would recommend the Watkins' *Natural Health Bible for Women* by Marilyn Glenville.

 Skin love

Prostaglandins can make your skin a bit more sensitive than usual. At the beginning of your cycle, your hormones are at their absolute lowest, producing less sebum. As a result, your face may feel a bit dry or look greyer than usual.

Try to treat your skin and your body gently during the inner winter. Keeping the skin moisturized with vitamin E products can help rehydrate the skin, strengthen the skin barrier and boost skin cell turnover.

 Exercise

This is the slowest phase of the menstrual cycle and now is the time to deeply honour this. There's no set way to exercise here, but perhaps be aware that endurance isn't one of winter's key skills; it may be difficult to keep up the pace during this inner season. That said, exercise releases endorphins, which are nature's pain relief, so it might be that some yoga or light cardio raises your mood and reduces cramping. It's lovely to wear loose clothing while doing this. Just be aware of any adjustments your body needs to make and only go with whatever feels right for you.

RESTORATIVE YOGA POSE

Ease back pain and relieve heavy, achy legs caused by period pain with this relaxing yoga pose. It is also great for relieving stress.

1. Sit on the floor. Place a cushion under your hips and gently put your legs up against a wall as you lie flat on your back.
2. Place your hips close to the wall or a little further away, depending on what's right for you.
3. Make sure your knees are comfortable, bending them if you prefer. Your arms can be in any position.
4. Rest here for ten minutes or so, but come out of the pose at any point that feels good.
5. When ready to move out of the pose, gently move away from the wall by drawing your knees to your chest, and rolling onto one side. Rise to your feet slowly and comfortably.

 Sleep on it

Nourish your body with some extra shut-eye whenever possible, during this time. Ideally, you would get at least seven hours of sleep during your period, but it's a good idea to work out what feels good for you. How much do you like to sleep to feel good? One way to think about this is to wonder how long you sleep on holiday as your benchmark. If it works out that you're not getting enough sleep during this phase, try to go to bed earlier, as often as possible.

The other thing to be aware of is how to join your values and health choices. Sleep is one of the most crucial aspects of being healthy, and our health is the most important thing there is. What takes you away from making good choices about your sleep? Is it Netflix, scrolling or other people, maybe? Aligning your health decisions with your values is key to sleeping better, and then having an easier period.

EMOTIONAL HEALING

The deep presence that inner winter brings can be incredibly rewarding. In winter, we can feel that we want to surrender to "something deeper". What might that be? Meeting our minds with curiosity and sensitivity can inspire some lightbulb moments, and we will explore this next.

Hoping to retreat during winter, when there are many external expectations to fulfil, can feel challenging. To fully explore this time, we need to welcome our nervous system on board, and breathwork can help with this (see below).

 Curiosity writing prompts

To fully let go during inner winter, we need to lovingly understand our limitations and what might be holding us back. Take some time to consider these questions:

- How do you experience your bleed?
- How open are you with others about your period?
- How do you feel when you're not busy?
- What's your relationship like with your job? E.g. Are you finishing on time and do you take on more than your role requires?
- Who takes most from you during inner winter?
- When do you tend to over-extend during this phase?
- What comes to mind when you think of the word "productive"?
- When are you tender with yourself?
- How have you nourished yourself in your other inner seasons this month?
- How do you feel about putting yourself first?

BREATHWORK: OCEAN BREATH

Ocean (or ujjayi) breath can help cultivate inner calm and regulate the nervous system, which is so helpful during inner winter. This breathwork can help you go inward and feel more in tune with the present moment.

1. If possible, close your eyes. If this feels too intense, try with your eyes open. Keep your lips together and breathe through your nose.
2. Slightly constrict the back of your throat, starting with an exhale, so that your breathing makes the sound of the sea (or slight snoring!).

3. When you're comfortable, do the same small throat constriction for the inhale. You should now sound a bit like Darth Vader.
4. Keep your inhale and exhale of equal lengths with long, slow breaths. Continue for about five minutes, if comfortable.
5. Come out of the practice gently when it feels right.

 ## Mindfulness: art therapy

Art induces a sense of meditation and surrender that the inner winter craves. This kind of creativity also improves anxiety, telling the brain that it's safe.

You will need:
- paper
- pens, pencils or paints
- scissors
- glue

1. Draw or paint all the things that pull you down in the world. This drawing doesn't have to look "good" and can take any form you like.
2. When you've finished, cut up the paper into little pieces.
3. On another piece of paper, draw the outline of a feather. Again, this doesn't need to look a certain way.
4. Glue or stick the cut-up pieces of paper onto your feather. Things can start to feel lighter now.
5. If you like, colour the paper using your pencils and pens with anything extra that inspires you to release.

Meditation: wisdom

In each of the meditation practices across the inner seasons, we have worked on paying attention to an emotional energy centre of the body. Here, we draw our focus to the top of our head or crown. The crown space represents connection and devotion.

In our inner winter, we get the chance to get "taken up with" a deep sense of consciousness. This connection to ourselves and others, whether alone or not, can be felt when we simply allow space for it.

You will need:
- candle, of your choice
- incense, of your choice

1. Find a spot at home to relax. Lay your candle and incense out in front of you, dim the lights and put on some relaxing music.
2. Slowly light the candle and incense. Breathe.
3. Raise your arms in a prayer position just above the top of your head. If this isn't possible for you, sit with a straight spine or a more restorative pose.
4. Simply listen. How does the area of the top of your head feel? What feels good and what feels stuck?
5. Be with this crown centre for as long as it feels OK.
6. If you like, imagine a white light flowing into the top of your head, clearing anything unwanted.
7. When you're ready, bring your attention back to the space you're in and open your eyes.
8. Gently blow out the flame of your candle and give thanks to your meditation practice.

Handling an over-talker in relationships

Have you noticed how everything suddenly seems louder and busier during your period? When all you want to do is be a bit useless for a few days (and I encourage it!), it can feel draining to be around someone who takes over the conversation or doesn't give you enough space to be your true self ... or just to *be*.

Over-talking can be due to nervousness or inadequacy, or a way to avoid deeper moments and keep things surface-level. Otherwise, it can be an effort to maintain control. How someone communicates speaks of their healing journey, and it helps to be aware of this when dealing with an over-talker. (Mansplaining is entirely different, and should never be tolerated!)

If your over-talker is a loved one or friend, my first tip is to make time for this person during inner spring or summer, when our tolerance and energy levels are higher. If avoidance isn't a real-life option, try these two hacks to prevent an emotional hangover and develop a sense of understanding about the issue:

- Take time away from everyone during inner winter to switch off from the outside world. Valuing self-care will help keep you rooted in what's important this week.
- Put a time limit on social exchanges beforehand and communicate your time boundaries. Having a few handy phrases such as, "circling back to what I was saying", or "I got a bit lost there" or "I'll just finish what I was saying" can be helpful, depending on who you are speaking with. Over-talking can be a symptom of ADHD or GAD (generalized anxiety disorder), so please be aware of this when making informed decisions about your communication.

Self-love: types of rest

Inner winter is the season of rest. Sleep, of course, is fundamental to wellbeing, but we also need other types of rest to feel fully restored. Rest isn't lazy or selfish (who taught us that?) – it's a vital and loving break for our nervous system.

- **Creative rest:** Being creative in whatever way feels good helps us engage with the moment and trust in the gorgeousness of life.
- **Emotional rest:** Releasing emotions in an aligned way creates a sense of inner honesty and deeper inner peace. Journalling and therapy are good examples.
- **Spiritual rest:** Connecting to the oneness of life helps us connect to something greater than our personal needs and wants.
- **Sensory rest:** Getting out in nature and dimming the noise of life leads to a calmer inner state.
- **Social rest:** Creating boundaries with emotionally draining people and staying connected to those who understand us brings about a fulfilling rest.
- **Mental rest:** Allowing your brain time to rest from never-ending activity helps with fatigue and focus.
- **Physical rest:** Relaxing our bodies from all the tension we carry around with us is a restorative way to truly rest.
- **Menstrual rest:** All of the above! We need pockets of every type of rest for us to navigate this time of deep surrender.

What types of rest are you seeking and what kinds are you lacking? How can you invite more rest into your world? Does any type of rest from the list above, really appeal to you? Take a moment now to think about how you can bring this into your life during inner winter (and at any time too!).

BIG BLEED

If you would like to know more about a concept known as the "big bleed", the ultimate restful menstrual experience, I would sincerely recommend the ground-breaking book, *Wild Power* by Alexandra Pope and Sjanie Wurlitzer. This means going "off the radar" during your period to fully experience the gifts and insights of the menstrual phase. It will take some planning, for example, taking time off work or arranging childcare. It's a total break from the outside world to be at one with your body.

SPIRITUAL HEALING

Inner winter is the birthplace of spiritual wisdom, total surrender and moments of absolute clarity, also known as claircognizance. Claircognizance is about "knowing things" without an explanation. Evolving our spiritual health through sacred practices can lead us deeper into personal insights and realizations. Let's look at a story to help us understand this concept.

FOLKTALE STORY: CERIDWEN

Ceridwen (Cerridwen or Caridwen) is known in Welsh folklore as the Crone goddess of prophecy, wisdom and transformation.

Watched by her white cats, Ceridwen created a potion in her infamous cauldron for her "monstrous" son, Morfran (or Avagduu), intending to transform him into a brilliant leader. After a year and a day, her brew was finally ready, only to be spilt by her servant, Gwion Bach, who was tending to this potion with an enormous spoon.

Outraged, Ceridwen chased Gwion, relentlessly. Both shapeshifting into many forms, Gwion's fate came to an end when he turned into a single grain of wheat, thinking he could escape her. Ceridwen ate the grain by transforming into a hen and the victory was hers. This seed took root in her body and Gwion (or Talieson as he was known) was reborn, later becoming a great bard to the leaders of his day.

Just like menstruation, Ceridwen brings us transformation whether we like it or not. She will force you to stop and surrender to her. Even if things aren't what we want or think we need, this Crone goddess will always know more. Eating away at the old life script, Ceridwen invites us to live differently now. Old ways grow stale while deeper discovery is resurrected.

In the pursuit of Gwion through many shapeshifting forms, we are reminded of the impermanence of life and the changing seasons of death and rebirth. Menstruation is like our inner death; a sacred pause before the rebirth in spring. In winter, we must sit in the gap to rebuild the ability to take on more in the next phase.

Living according to the unique power of each changing inner season allows your "you-ness" to flow through you without the usual self-imposed limits. You are a source of power at every corner.

Self-expression: niksen

Self-expression is, in its essence, embracing who we are. We do this by actively engaging in something. In this season, there is no better way to "do" self-expression than to simply do nothing. Niksen is the Dutch term for doing nothing, and it's about exactly what it says on the tin. Doing nothing helps us reframe what it means to rest and helps us to feel anchored in the moment. Here's how:

- Turn off all screens.
- Do nothing for a while. A "while" looks like anything that feels good to you.
- You might like to sit watching the rain pattering on the window, or the clouds float by.
- You might like to watch a pet snooze.
- You might like to go on a purposeless walk.
- There is no outcome, no agenda and no dopamine hit to be chased by being active. Simply be!

 ## Crystals: oneness

With its healing energies, moonstone is our inner winter special gem. Connected to the divine feminine, moonstone invites us to trust moments of deep intuition and honour our cyclicality. Moonstone can help us feel at peace with ourselves and the world around us – a oneness.

Oneness is a difficult sensation to explain, and only one that we can understand through direct contact, but it's a state of being that just is.

Moving beyond the confines of the self helps us open the door to a feeling of oneness. Moonstone can help unlock this connection to the universe. Wearing your moonstone or placing it onto your third eye centre (middle of forehead) while meditating (or doing nothing) connects us to the web of life.

Womb ritual: blood offering

A few years ago, I received the 13th Rite of the Munay Ki from a healer. This is a beautiful transmission connected to the divine feminine and the 13 moons of the year, helping people clear wounds from their womb centres. It was originally gifted to Marcela Lobos by a group of medicine women in South America who brought it to the Western world with permission. The rite is:

"The womb is not a place to store fear and pain. The womb is to create and give birth to life."

For 13 cycles after receiving the rite, I was told to offer my blood back to the earth to continue the path of womb healing. Here, I got to understand blood magick. If you ever get a chance to receive this rite from a local practitioner, I'd wholeheartedly champion this.

You can, of course, take part in a blood offering at any point during menstruation as a way to create a ritualistic relationship with your womb centre. This breaks down the stigma of periods and brings you closer to your body.

The menstrual cycle is at the heart of our lineages. Without it, there would be no people. When we menstruate, we connect to our ancestors, and when we offer this blood to the earth, we intimately connect with the power of nature and the divine feminine. It's a reciprocal exchange of energy, as menstrual blood contains healing stem cells and nutrients that the soil loves. Try this during your period, during your inner winter.

You will need:
- period pants, reusable pad or menstrual cup
- small bowl
- paper and paint brushes, if you choose

1. Soak your period pants or reusable pad (without soap) in water and squeeze them out, collecting the red water in a small bowl. Or collect your blood in the menstrual cup and dilute it in some water.
2. Pour the red water onto soil, perhaps in your garden, woodland or into a houseplant pot.
3. Feel free to say something personal during your blood offering. The winter affirmations below work well here.
4. You can take this offering further by using it in a spell to amplify the magic or using some of the sacred water to paint and get creative. Feel free to paint on your body, if you choose.

 ## Winter affirmations

These affirmations are here to let you off the hook. There's no motive here other than to surrender. Let's just give in to it all.

I see the divine feminine that lives within me.
I release control and doubt.
I allow spiritual insight to unfold within me.
I trust in the sweetness of existence.
I am being paced by something bigger than myself.

*I am at peace with myself and the world around me.
I am made of stardust and radiate the deepest love.
It's safe to sink into the moment.*

 ## Essential oil: clary sage

Clary sage is lovely during menstruation as it helps with cramp pain and also helps regulate the nervous system. Some aromatherapists think clary sage can help to plug us into our spiritual insights by enhancing dreamwork and deeper intuition.

Inner winter is the season of dreaming. Dreams are thought to be representations of our unconscious mind. They can also be manifestations of our spiritual powers, revealing how we can use our cosmic abilities in everyday life. When we bleed, it's said the veil between the material and the spirit world is thin, allowing us to receive divine wisdom more freely. Clary sage can give us glimpses into our spiritual lessons on this planet.

There are many ways to use oils; one way to use clary sage to open up intuition is to add a few drops to a bowl of steaming water, place a towel over your head and breathe in the steam to remedy your mind, body and soul. Alternatively, add a drop or two to your pillow at night.

 ## Cosmic ceremony: enoughness

Spending time with other people who get the magnitude of this season's gifts – even if they are not menstruating at the same time – feels beautifully therapeutic and cathartic. Knowing that, beyond period stigma and non-stop schedules, there are people who connect deeply to their cyclical bodies, can create bonds of togetherness like nothing else.

How do we seek togetherness in today's world? Now, belonging to something bigger than ourselves takes the form of going after "the next hyped thing". This distracts us from our enoughness and hooks us into the need to have more to be more. Striving is necessary, but so is gratitude.

When we are like others, we feel included. To be part of something makes the world go round. I like the idea of a different kind of togetherness; one where we remind each other of the inherent power that resides within us all.

Here, we are going to gather in a "red tent". This is a supportive space created for women by women to reflect and connect with each other. It can be in a room, or an outdoor space.

You will need:
- soft cushions, throws and candles, of any colour
- relaxing music

1. Create a sacred space using your gathered items. Dim the lights, turn your phones on silent, light some candles, play music and sit in a circle on soft cushions.
2. Take some time to reflect on this stage in your cycle, whether menstruating or not. Give everyone the time and space to be heard if they choose to share. Perhaps you can ask questions such as:

- What do you know to be true about yourself?
- How is your insight directing you?
- What do you love about yourself?
- What do you want to let go of?

3. You can close the sacred space in whatever way feels right for you all. This is a time of just being in the moment and going with whatever flows.

INNER WINTER AND THE OTHER CYCLES

Lean in further, lovelies, as we take our cyclical voyage further. Let's journey into how your inner seasons can be impacted by the three other ways of living cyclically. Our inner menstrual seasons may recalibrate a little depending on where we sit in our lunar, seasonal and life cycles.

 Winter and the lunar cycle

We explore the red moon and white moon cycles further in this section. Some ancient cultures may have used these terms to explore the spiritual meaning behind the lunar and menstrual connection. How might your inner winter alter according to the phases of the moon?

Winter and the new moon

There's a special kind of sorcery to this cyclical blend. Two quiet powerhouses, winter and the new moon can work together to help you start afresh. Bleeding at the time of the new moon and ovulating with the full moon is known as the white moon cycle. This bleeding pattern echoes the natural rhythm of the lunar phases. The earth is thought to be at its most fertile during the full moon because of the extra moonlight. We, as women, are at our most fertile during ovulation and this is a time of open-heartedness and reflection. The white moon archetype is the Mother, and right now we're being called to nurture ourselves and explore our softer energies.

Winter and the waxing moon

Bleeding with the waxing moon is known as the pink moon cycle. Experiencing your inner winter during this lunar phase can symbolize a time of transition and growth. Waxing moon intentions can feel softer while menstruating. If not, try slowing down the waxing moon's energy to the pace of your inner winter's intuitive wisdom. This can help you avoid any dissonance. Try checking in with your values more deeply (see page 70) and make time for rest so intuition can come to the fore.

Winter and the full moon

When you menstruate on the full moon (and ovulate with the new moon), we call this the red cycle. It's thought there is an extra layer of inner potential that helps you navigate winter from a deeply empowered place. This can help you turn negativity into creative action, inspiring others as you do so. Facing our wounds during the full moon with winter's tendency to resist surrender can feel jarring; remember to sit with the necessary pockets of letting go that menstruation requires.

Winter and the waning moon

Bleeding as the moon starts to disappear from the sky brings a beautiful energy of reflection. Drawing everything to a close, this fusion sees a move away from the sounds of the material world to a deeply heightened intuition. If this time feels too deep, look at how you sit with the concept of rest and retreat. There's a silence to inner winter and the waning moon that may feel too ruminative. If so, reach out to your fellow witches if things feel all too inward.

MOON SPELL FOR RETREAT

Winter asks us to be with the simplicity of what's real, despite our round-the-clock commitments. Creating an intention of deep rest can be a powerful way to honour the sacredness of your bleed, regardless of the lunar phase.

You will need:
- charcoal disc
- lighter
- heatproof dish
- dried lavender

1. Open a window. Cleanse the space you want to rest in by carefully lighting the edge of the charcoal disc with your lighter, and immediately putting it into your heatproof dish.
2. When the charcoal disc turns grey, sprinkle a small pinch of your dried lavender onto it.
3. Hold your dish and gently circle the smoke in clockwise movements around the space, while walking around the room. The lavender will purify the area as the smoke cleanses away any negative energy.

4. Say this incantation three times out loud:

   "I call a slowness to my pace. I let go of the never-ending chase. Three times, rest infuses this sacred place."

5. When you're ready, put your heatproof dish somewhere safe, let the remaining smoke die off and rest in your cleansed space for a while.

❄. Winter and the yearly cycle

Each of the ways of living cyclically can influence each other. Our inner winter experience can alter depending on what season of the year we find ourselves within. Let's steal a look at how your inner winter may transform throughout the year.

Inner winter and yearly spring

The rise of the external season and the fall of the inner season may result in challenges as you navigate the contradicting energies. Our inner cycles are much shorter than our yearly ones, so we have opportunities to feel more in tune with cyclical rhythms later in the month. The potential of this cyclical blend rests in the ability to approach spring with a deeper appreciation of what you want to change or rise within you. Inner winter's sagacity can help you see yearly spring as a beautiful cauldron of possibility.

Inner winter and yearly summer

As the year heats up, we are being called to our deepest fullness, and when we menstruate, we are being invited to retreat. A beautiful paradox. Here, you can experience the richness of your bleed with the absoluteness and saturation that summer brings. Try not to get carried away with the outwardness of the summer energies, giving your body the time and space to rest.

Inner winter and yearly autumn

Both energies urge us to go underground, and we often need to turn the lights down to make sense of what lies beneath the surface. Now can feel like an easier few days as the external season supports the menstrual call to retreat. However, this time can also feel unforgiving, especially toward the end of the year, when the nights draw in and our capacity to be effortful shrinks. We may feel like we can't get as much done, which plays into underlying feelings of inadequacy. Your self-care sessions to restore dips in confidence are your ally during any energetic clashes.

Inner winter and yearly winter

The void is upon us. Relishing the nothingness can feel restful and transformative, or it may feel all too overcast out there. Menstruating during winter is an opportunity to avoid stuffing the empty gap with uncertainty and control, and simply being with whatever comes to you, and from you. But being unproductive, even for a few short days, can feel like a killer in a world where continual productivity is approved of. There will be plenty of time for purpose later this month, so dip into "the slow" for this brief moment in time.

 ## Winter and the life cycle

Your inner winter can be experienced differently depending on which life phase you're currently enjoying.

Winter and Maiden

The archetype of the Maiden represents hope, vitality and high energy. Your menstrual energy, however, may feel dark, heavy and unproductive. Fusing the two energies is supported by your self-awareness. Being aware that nothing is permanent and that it's possible to hold both the light and the shadow will allow the descent into menstruation to feel easier. We have to surrender a little during our periods, even during our high-energy years, otherwise we'll end up feeling overwhelmed.

Winter and Mother

You can use your nurturing life cycle energies to tend to your tired body during menstruation. It may also be an opportunity to work on ancestral Mother wounds hiding from view (see page 18). There's a loving feeling that encompasses both the inner winter and the archetypal Mother, but let go of the need to "get the job done", otherwise, you may burn out come inner spring.

Winter and Wild Woman

Spiritual insights can intensify with age and experience, so you may find your inner winter feels more perceptive during your Wild Woman years. Using these spiritual insights to direct your path in life is a beautiful bonus to your cyclical journey. You may also find that things feel a bit chaotic as your periods change during your peri-menopausal years. Keeping your oestrogen and progesterone balanced with optimum nutrition and low stress is a good recipe for maintaining stability.

Winter and Crone

The Crone works out who they are and who they're not without the support of a cycle. Some of you have crossed the threshold into the exquisite power and gifts of the Crone, and I can only dream of what this divine state of consciousness feels like. I have nothing more to say as you are wiser than I can only imagine.

Enjoying a slower pace during inner winter helps us put our worries to rest. In the first half of our menstrual cycle, we build towards showing up to the world, peaking with the brightness of inner summer. When autumn calls, we're ready to confront the shadow, peeling away old, unhelpful beliefs. This seasonal work gets us ready to meet the gifts of inner winter. When the quiet of winter draws you into yourself, you're at one with your essence, dissolving the need to be anything other than your truest self.

FINAL THOUGHTS

I won't say goodbye as it's never really the end. As things come to a close, we begin again. This is the cycle of life: death and rebirth, winter and spring, old and new. A process so spectacular and limitless, it's beyond measure. Rather, we flow. Flow through each cycle while each season loyally holds space for us to transform and renew.

Whether it's the last page of a book or the last days of our cycle, fresh beginnings are on the horizon. What new experiences will you relish as a result of reading these chapters? What new insights will you bring into your self-discovery journey? How do you plan to take care of yourself moving forward? How will your life transform now you're living in alignment with the seasons and the moon?

I hope there have been lightbulb moments, even on the cloudy days, that have helped you gain a different perspective on life. I have created this book for you to come back to ... or come home to, again and again. There's much to integrate, and it's a process. I am forever grateful for your time and wisdom on this path together. Each turn of the wheel, each phase of the moon, each stage of life and each season of the menstrual cycle, takes you closer to your truth, one cyclical step at a time.

Our four cycles remind us that everything changes. When we flow with, instead of fighting against, our natural patterns, we learn to navigate life more beautifully. Balance, resilience, rest, vulnerability, strength, power and, most of all, joy. Joy is felt in the simple act of living in this world. And what an exquisite place it is to call home.

FURTHER READING

Period poverty

In the UK, 10 per cent of girls can't afford to buy menstrual products and are therefore missing school. Breaking the silencing around this and supporting charities such as *Bloody Good Period* can help combat this serious issue. In the US, 20 per cent reported experiencing this issue every month.

Trans and non-binary menstruators

If you would like to expand your knowledge of trans and non-binary menstruators, please go to the *International Journal of Transgender Health* to learn more.

Part 1: Life cycle

Blackie, Sharon, *Hagitude: Reimagining the Second Half of Life*, September Publishing, Tewkesbury, 2023

Chollet, Mona, *In Defence of Witches: Why women are still on trial*, Picador, London, 2022, p.172

Estés, Clarissa Pinkola, *Women Who Run With The Wolves*, Rider, London, 2008, p.246 and p.388

Gray, Miranda, *Red Moon: Understanding and using the creative, sexual and spiritual gifts of the menstrual cycle*, Dancing Eve, 2009, p.170

Harlow, Siobán D, et al., "Disparities in Reproductive Aging and Midlife Health between Black and White Women", *Women's Midlife*

Health, 8(3), 2022, womensmidlifehealthjournal.biomedcentral.com/articles/10.1186/s40695-022-00073-y

Lynch, Jackie, *The Happy Menopause: Smart Nutrition to Help You Flourish*, Watkins, London, 2020

Marchiano, Lisa, *Motherhood: Facing and Finding Yourself*, Sounds True, Louisville, 2021, Preface

Owen, Lara, *Her Blood Is Gold*, Archive Publishing, Shaftesbury 2008, Preface XII

Part 2: Seasonal cycle

Ammar, A, Trabelsi, K, Boukhris O, Bouaziz B, Müller P, M Glenn J, Bott NT, Müller N, Chtourou H, Driss T, Hökelmann A, "Effects of Polyphenol-Rich Interventions on Cognition and Brain Health in Healthy Young and Middle-Aged Adults: Systematic review and meta-analysis", *Journal of Clinical Medicine*, 9(5), 2020

Campaign to end loneliness, www.campaigntoendloneliness.org/facts-and-statistics/

Pretani Wisdom Traditions, "Imbolc 2024", Pretani Wisdom Traditions, 2024, pretani.uk/Blog-Posts/Imbolc-2024/

Part 3: Lunar cycle

Casiraghi, L, et al., "Moonstruck Sleep: Synchronization of human sleep with the moon cycle under field conditions", *Science Advances*, 7(5), 2021

Feenstra S, et al, "Contextualizing the Impostor "Syndrome"", *Front Psychol*, 11(405), 13 Nov 2020, www.ncbi.nlm.nih.gov/pmc/articles/PMC7703426/

Part 4: Menstrual cycle

Basso, J, McHale, A, Ende, V, Oberlin, D, Suzuki, W, "Brief, Daily Meditation Enhances Attention, Memory, Mood, and Emotional Regulation in Non-experienced Meditators". *Behavioral Brain Research, 356, 2019*

Blackie, Sharon, *If Women Rose Rooted: A Life Changing Journey to Authenticity and Belonging*, September Publishing, Tewkesbury, 2019, p. 131

Digdon, N, Koble, A, "Effects of Constructive Worry, Imagery Distraction, and Gratitude Interventions on Sleep Quality: A pilot trial", *Applied Psychology: Health and Well-Being*, 3(2), 2011

Hertel, J, König, J, Homuth, G, *et al.*, "Evidence for Stress-like Alterations in the HPA-Axis in Women Taking Oral Contraceptives". *Scientific Reports*, 7(1), 2017

Holdcroft, A, "Gender bias in research: how does it affect evidence based medicine?" *Journey of the Royal Society of Medicine*, 100(1), 2007

Holt, N. J., Furbert, L., Sweetingham, E, "Cognitive and Affective Benefits of Coloring: Two randomized controlled crossover studies", *Art Therapy*, 36(4), 2019, pp.200–208.

Le'Nise Brothers, *You Can Have a Better Period: A Practical Guide to Calmer and Less Painful Periods*, Watkins Publishing, London, 2022

Lobos, Marcela, *The Rite of the Womb*, 2024, marcelalobos.com/the-rite-of-the-womb/

Martínez-Fortuny, N, Alonso-Calvete, A, Da Cuña-Carrera, I, Abalo-Núñez, R, "Menstrual Cycle and Sport Injuries: A systematic review", *International Journal of Environmental Research and Public Health*, 20(4), 2023

Pope, Alexandra and Wurlitzer, Sjanie Hugo, *Wild Power: Discover the Magic of Your Menstrual Cycle and Awaken the Feminine Path to Power*, Hay House, Carlsbad, 2017

Rahbar N, Asgharzadeh N, Ghorbani R, "Effect of Omega-3 Fatty Acids on Intensity of Primary Dysmenorrhea", *International Journal of Gynecology & Obstetrics*, 117(1), 2012

Roney, J, Simmons, Z, "Hormonal Predictors of Sexual Motivation in Natural Menstrual Cycles", *Hormones and Behavior*, 63(4), 2013

Saint-Jean, M, Khammari, A, Seite, S, Moyal, D, Dreno, B, "Characteristics of Premenstrual Acne Flare-up and Benefits of a Dermocosmetic Treatment: a double-blind randomised trial", *European Journal of Dermatology*, 27(2), 2017

Sudimac S, Sale V, Kühn S, "How Nature Nurtures: Amygdala activity decreases as the result of a one-hour walk in nature", *Molecular Psychiatry*, 27(11), 2022

ACKNOWLEDGEMENTS

I'm so blessed and grateful to everyone who has raised me up and taught me something special along the way.

In particular, I want to thank my family for their unending support; my gals for their unending wisdom; my Aluna Moon partnership and our community on Insight Timer; and my many clients and colleagues over the years. Thanks to the University of Reading, and those who mentored me there, yoga the RNOH (The Royal National Orthopaedic Hospital) and the staff that do an amazing job there and *Happiful* Magazine, for being understanding when I became unwell and for teaching me new writing skills, amongst all the other things.

Becki Bond, for inviting me to Clio Wood's book launch where I met Ella, for running a beady eye over the manuscript and for being you. Katie Flaxman for helping me figure out my proposal, talk myths with me and make me a better writer by being a far better writer than I'll ever be. And for every lady in my village that helped me in some way with this book. Jenni Benzer for helping me with commas and for being an ongoing literary inspiration.

And especially the team at Watkins! Ella for taking a chance on me and for walking the tightrope of letting me "get on with it" and guiding me so perfectly. Emma and Sneha for capturing the essence of the book with lovely designs. Brittany for bringing this book to fruition wonderfully, moving the manuscript forward and being so positive in the process. Becky, for organizing the structure and managing the tone beautifully, being so incredibly knowledgeable in the area of wellbeing. Watkins, you all made the book simply *flow*.

INDEX

Note: page numbers in bold refer to illustrations